A Developmental Model of Borderline Personality Disorder

Understanding Variations in Course and Outcome

A Developmental Model of Borderline Personality Disorder

Understanding Variations in Course and Outcome

Patricia Hoffman Judd, Ph.D.
Clinical Professor of Psychiatry
University of California, San Diego, School of Medicine;
Program Director, Outpatient Psychiatric Services
University of California, San Diego,
San Diego, California

Thomas H. McGlashan, M.D.
Professor of Psychiatry
Yale University School of Medicine
Yale Psychiatric Institute
New Haven, Connecticut

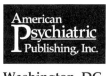

Washington, DC
London, England

Note: The authors have worked to ensure that all information in this book is accurate at the time of publication and consistent with general psychiatric and medical standards, and that information concerning drug dosages, schedules, and routes of administration is accurate at the time of publication and consistent with standards set by the U. S. Food and Drug Administration and the general medical community. As medical research and practice continue to advance, however, therapeutic standards may change. Moreover, specific situations may require a specific therapeutic response not included in this book. For these reasons and because human and mechanical errors sometimes occur, we recommend that readers follow the advice of physicians directly involved in their care or the care of a member of their family.

Manufactured in the United States of America on acid-free paper
07   06   05   04   03   5   4   3   2   1
First Edition

Typeset in Adobe's Palatino and Goudy

American Psychiatric Publishing, Inc.
1400 K Street, N.W.
Washington, DC 20005
www.appi.org

Library of Congress Cataloging-in-Publication Data
Judd, Patricia Hoffman, 1946–
    A developmental model of borderline personality disorder : understanding variations in course and outcome / Patricia Hoffman Judd, Thomas H. McGlashan.—1st ed.
        p. ; cm.
    Includes bibliographical references and index.
    ISBN 0-88048-515-9 (alk. paper)
    1. Borderline personality disorder—Etiology. 2. Borderline personality disorder—Treatment. 3. Borderline personality disorder—Case studies. I. McGlashan, Thomas H., 1941–   . II. Title.
    [DNLM: 1. Borderline Personality Disorder—therapy—Case Report. 2. Treatment Outcome—Case Report. WM 190 J92d 2003]
    RC569.5.B67 J834 2003
    616.85′85206—dc21

                                                                          2002027686

British Library Cataloguing in Publication Data
A CIP record is available from the British Library.

In memory of Rusty Bullard, M.D.,
Director of Chestnut Lodge Hospital from 1974 to 1994

With thanks to the patients, trainees, and my colleagues
over the years at UCSD Gifford Clinic—P.H.J.

With thanks to the patients and staff of
Chestnut Lodge Hospital—T.H.M.

Contents

I
Etiology

II
Variations in Course and Outcome:
Case Histories

III
Treatment

Introduction

This book is designed for clinicians interested in understanding and treating patients with borderline personality disorder (BPD) in both public mental health and private practice settings. The book is based on the authors' combined clinical, supervisory, and research experience over the past 30 years and a detailed study of the BPD patients included in the Chestnut Lodge Follow-Up Study described in Chapter 2.

In the late 1980s, we embarked on a project to elucidate the course and outcome of BPD through intensive case study of the rich clinical information available through the Chestnut Lodge study. Over the subsequent decade, the project lay dormant for long periods as we pursued other professional and personal activities on opposite coasts interspersed with revisions and resubmissions in response to suggestions by American Psychiatric Press peer reviewers. When the book was approved for publication, a whole decade's worth of new research had been conducted and required incorporation. We were pleasantly surprised to learn that, on careful review, the research provided empirical support for much of our original thinking on the disorder. In addition, the growing body of research conducted on maltreated children added immensely to our understanding of developmental course and outcome.

Out of this lengthy incubation period emerged a developmental model of etiology that promised to elucidate the enormous heterogeneity in BPD course and outcome and to inform treatment. Thus, we embarked on our final revision, and what started as a descriptive book on course and outcome was transformed into a theory-driven elaboration of etiology, course, and outcome illustrated by four prototypical cases and followed by a discussion of treatment implications.

Considerable pessimism still surrounds the treatment of BPD despite convincing empirical evidence that borderline patients improve with treatment and time. Even with these outcome findings and the availability of well-elaborated treatment approaches (described in Chapter 7: "Universal Features of Treatment") and a wide variety of psychopharmacological strategies, BPD patients remain underserved, have their treatment prematurely terminated, or are made worse by treatment systems that are inadequately designed to serve and help them. Social service, health, alcohol and drug treatment, and criminal justice settings also can be greatly impacted because of a similar lack of understanding.

A main goal of the book is to present BPD in all its variations through four cases that are representative of its range of severity, treatment responsiveness, and long-term outcome. Another major goal of the book is to provide a theoretical framework that tries to account for the puzzling, provocative, frustrating, and often frightening interpersonal behaviors that BPD patients exhibit in order to increase the clinician's empathy and ability to maintain an effective treatment alliance. Rather than provide a treatment manual, we offer a perspective on why various treatment approaches from varying theoretical perspectives can be effective and what BPD patients need from psychosocial treatment in order to improve or sustain functioning. We also hope that our work will function as a beginning synthesis for the large and ever-growing body of research and clinical literature on children and adults with BPD and perhaps provide some direction for more integrated future inquiry.

In Part I, we describe a multidimensional and integrated etiological model of BPD that incorporates developmental theory, attachment research, and research on maltreated children with genetic and biological investigations, neuropsychological findings, family studies, and long-term outcome studies of adult BPD patients. In Part II, we provide an overview of the Chestnut Lodge Follow-Up Study and other outcome studies and present four prototypical cases that represent a continuum from moderate impairment with good outcome to severe impairment with poor outcome. In Part III, we apply the developmental model and case histories to a discussion of treatment and its essential features and recurrent issues and themes.

For many readers new to the mental health field, the treatment experience of these patients will serve as an education in the history of psychological treatments in the United States. At the time the women herein described were patients at Chestnut Lodge, asylum and psychotherapy, with the occasional use of sedative-hypnotics, insulin shock therapy, electroconvulsive therapy (ECT), or ice packs, were considered state-of-the-art treatment. Although aspects of the treatment seem primitive and at times barbaric by today's standards, the modalities used were accepted practice at the time.

The criteria for a diagnosis of BPD as described in the American Psychiatric Association's *Diagnostic and Statistical Manual of Mental Disorders,* Fourth Edition, Text Revision (DSM-IV-TR), includes a pervasive pattern of instability of interpersonal relationships, self-image, and emotions and marked impulsivity. This pattern begins by early adulthood and presents in a variety of contexts. Individuals with this diagnosis engage in unstable and intense relationships, fear abandonment, and have difficulty being alone. They exhibit self-damaging behaviors, such as promiscuity, substance abuse, recurrent suicidal behavior, or self-mutilating behavior, and express intense anger or rage that seems out of proportion to situations. BPD patients also experience dissociation and a variety of other cognitive problems and, under stress, can become paranoid or develop other brief psychotic states. As with all personality disorders, the behavior of BPD patients deviates markedly from the expectations of our culture and is inflexible and pervasive across a broad range of personal and social situations.

The authors want to thank the patients, clinicians, and researchers who worked at Chestnut Lodge Hospital for making this work possible. We tried to walk in the shoes of both patients and clinicians to understand their struggle. We hope that our rendering of their work together pays tribute to the courage and heroic efforts of the patients to live and adapt and of the clinicians to persevere and understand. Finally, we hope that this work provides a guiding light and encouragement to those suffering from, treating, and conducting research on the disorder.

Chestnut Lodge Hospital closed its doors since this book began and ended a unique era in the history of the residential treatment of mental illness. The sweeping changes in pharmacotherapy, the emphasis on least restrictive settings for treatment, and the application of managed care strategies contributed to the hospital's demise. We hope that this book might also reinstate the value of long-term asylum and village in our mental health treatment systems.

The patients who participated in the Chestnut Lodge Follow-Up Study gave verbal and written consent for inclusion in the study. They were told that the information they gave would be published as group data or disguised case reports and that their identification would remain confidential. Families and/or the last treating psychiatrist were interviewed for patients who were deceased at the time of follow-up. This was acceptable practice in 1980 according to Chestnut Lodge Hospital and the National Institute of Mental Health, which funded the study. Publication of clinical case reports was considered ethical as long as identifying information was removed and/or sufficiently disguised. Such efforts have been made to maintain the anonymity of the patients included in these case histories.

Acknowledgments

We acknowledge the former Chestnut Lodge Hospital and Research Institute; the University of California, San Diego, School of Medicine Department of Psychiatry; and Yale Psychiatric Research and Medical School for support during preparation of this book.

Etiology

An Integrated
Developmental Model

…it is not news that we live in a world
Where beauty is suddenly ruined
And has its own routines. We are often far
From home in a dark town, and our griefs
Are difficult to translate into a language
Understood by others.

Charlie Smith, "The Meaning of Birds"

John, a handsome, blue-eyed, 18-year-old student, calls his care coordinator and after an initial tense silence states tersely that he is planning to jump off the walking bridge within view of her office window. Within minutes John appears on the bridge. The care coordinator calls the police psychiatric emergency team and runs toward the bridge. At each step her heart pounds, as she fears that John will jump.

Bill, a 34-year-old married man and father of two, calls his therapist and tells him he has a gun to his head and is playing Russian roulette. Bill warns the therapist that if he calls the police he has an escape route planned and will never be found. The gun clicks once over the phone and Bill hangs up. The therapist frantically calls 911 and summons the police to Bill's home.

The behaviors of the patients above are examples of the behaviors of patients with borderline personality disorder (BPD) that challenge mental health professionals. These behaviors and the emotions they evoke have made BPD patients one of the most researched and discussed patient groups in the mental health profession. Despite considerable study, the disorder continues to perplex and challenge.

John was unable to engage in ongoing psychotherapy and, after numerous brief hospitalizations and trials on multiple medications, shot and killed himself on the lawn of his pastor's church at the age of 25. Bill, with long-term psychotherapy and medications, was able to maintain his marriage, raise his children, and work, albeit with difficulty. This wide variation in course and outcome has also been one of the puzzling aspects of the disorder.

In this book, we attempt to provide an integrated etiological model of BPD that explains its clinical phenomenology, describes the broad variations in course and outcome, and informs treatment. This model, outlined in Figure 1–1, is based on a transactional approach in which genetic, biological, and environmental forces influence one another and make reciprocal contributions to developmental outcomes (Sameroff and Chandler 1975). The model integrates cumulative evidence from genetic and biological investigations, studies of maltreated children, and neuropsychological, clinical, and long-term outcome studies with theories of personality, development, and attachment.

We propose that the individual who develops the borderline disorder is born into the world with a range of neurobehavioral vulnerabilities that are amplified and exaggerated by environmental factors. Vulnerabilities, as defined by Cowan et al. (1996), can be conceptualized as conditions or processes associated with an increased risk for negative outcomes when combined with another vulnerability or during times of increased stress.

The central foundation for this theory is the organizational model of normal development, which posits that normal development is a progression from diffuse and undifferentiated states to states of more organized complexity (Cicchetti and Schneider-Rosen 1984, 1986; Sroufe 1979). In this model, the child's development is marked by the differentiation and hierarchical organization of interdependent competencies in the emotional, social, and cognitive arenas. Developmental accomplishments occur within the matrix of the attachment system and continue to be shaped by the environment throughout life. They are continually reintegrated with subsequent accomplishments. Each successive adaptation is a product both of new experiences and of development to that point. Psychopathology emerges largely because of a lack of integration of the many competencies that underlie adaptation at various developmental stages (Cicchetti and Schneider-Rosen 1984, 1986; Sroufe and Rutter 1984).

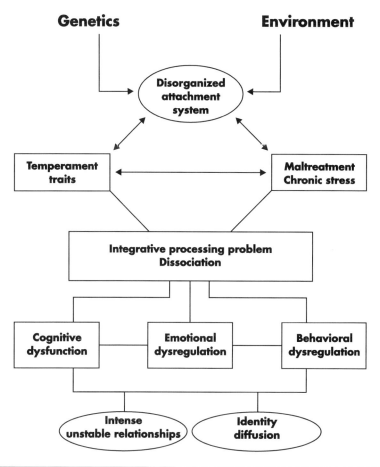

FIGURE 1–1.   Integrated model of borderline personality disorder.

The neurodevelopmental vulnerabilities that underlie BPD include a possible genetic predisposition (Torgersen 2000; Torgersen et al. 2000) and prenatal and postnatal problems that express themselves through structural abnormalities in the brain and disorders of neurobehavioral systems. The environment, consisting of parents, extended family, friends, and community systems, aggravates and amplifies these vulnerabilities through various forms of maltreatment. Adverse life events further weaken the family's ability to provide sufficient nurturance, guidance, structure, and support to help the child compensate for and remediate these problems.

Both neurodevelopmental vulnerabilities and environmental factors are mediated through the attachment system that serves as the central pathway for the development of the disorder. Neurodevelopmental vulnerabilities are expressed through temperament, traits, and information-processing abilities. Temperamental characteristics and traits associated with BPD include characteristics such as high novelty seeking, high harm avoidance, and low reward dependence (Cloninger 1998) and traits such as high neuroticism and gregariousness, low straightforwardness, low compliance in social relations, and low achievement striving (Widiger et al. 1994). These temperamental characteristics and traits are also described as *impulsive aggression* and *affective instability* (Siever and Davis 1991). The cognitive-processing problems found in individuals with BPD (Carpenter et al. 1993; Judd and Ruff 1993; O'Leary et al. 1991; Swirsky-Sacchetti et al. 1993) interfere with the integration of emotional and sensorimotor information into interpersonal memory systems. These information-processing problems underlie and maintain dissociation among memory systems. As a result, an insecure disorganized attachment pattern, characterized by multiple unintegrated and dissociated models, develops.

Within this framework, the clinical phenomenology of the disorder can be understood as a manifestation of complex developmental deficits and integrative failures or a complex developmental (socio-emotive-dyssocial) disorder, as is now being suggested for the borderline disorder in children (Ad-Dab'Bagh and Greenfield 2001; Lincoln et al. 1998; Towbin et al. 1993). This disorder is characterized by multiple dissociated states of mind or modes of attachment that lead to unstable interpersonal relationships and identity confusion and delayed or distorted cognitive, emotional, and behavioral development. Deviation spreads along so many developmental lines because the developmental process is set off course beginning in infancy, and when the disorder is untreated, the process persists in that direction throughout childhood and adolescence and into adulthood.

On the basis of this model, the clinical phenomenology can be organized as follows:

I. Insecure and disorganized/disoriented attachment with fluctuations between preoccupied and dismissing models

    a. Unstable and intense interpersonal relationships
    b. Identity disturbance
    c. Intimacy impediment

II. Cognitive processing dysfunction

    a. Severe dissociation
    b. Impaired metacognitive monitoring
    c. Denial

　　　d. Splitting
　　　e. Stress-related paranoid states/projection
　　　f. Stress-related psychotic states
　III. Emotional dysregulation
　　　a. Affective instability and hypersensitivity
　　　b. Numbness
　　　c. Chronic feelings of emptiness
　　　d. Inappropriate, intense anger
　IV. Behavioral dysregulation
　　　a. Reenacting instead of remembering
　　　b. Frantic efforts to avoid real or imagined abandonment
　　　c. Impulsivity in at least two areas that are self-damaging
　　　d. Recurrent suicidal behavior, gestures, or threats
　　　e. Self-mutilating behaviors

We will now elaborate on the primary components of the model as summarized above and outlined in Figure 1–1 and attempt to explicate how these factors might interact with one another in the course of development. Our overall emphasis is to understand etiology in terms that will explain variations in long-term course and elucidate treatment. The reader is reminded that the model is dynamic and nonlinear. However, for purposes of presentation, these factors must be presented in linear fashion.

PERSONALITY

To understand a personality disorder, we must first place it in the context of general personality theory. *Personality* refers to a dynamic organization of the psychobiological systems that modulate adaptation to experience (Cloninger 1987). *Temperament*—the biological predispositions or automatic responses to emotional stimuli that influence and shape personality—forms the foundation for any model of personality disorder. Temperament is considered to be 50% heritable, stable over time, emotion based, and relatively uninfluenced by sociocultural learning (Goldsmith et al. 1987). Temperament, which refers to our basic emotionality, is perceptually based and well developed at an early age (Cloninger 1994, 1995). It appears to correspond to systems in the brain, especially the limbic system and striatum and their corresponding neurotransmitters or neuromodulaters, that are related to habit or procedural learning and that include behavioral activation, inhibition, reinforcement, and social attachment (Cloninger 1998).

Personality traits, which can be defined as enduring "dimensions of individual differences in tendencies to show consistent patterns of thoughts, feelings, and actions" (McCrae and Costa 1990, p. 23), can also be understood as manifestations of underlying genetic and biological forces. Extreme or excessive expressions of personality traits are hypothesized by some to define personality disorders and by others to define risk for personality disorders.

GENETIC AND BIOLOGICAL FACTORS

In this section, we present a sampling of the findings, from both adult and child studies, regarding the genetic and biological basis for BPD. We include evidence from studies on maltreated children, as we think these findings are highly relevant to an understanding of the disorder.

The genetic and biological investigation into BPD is still in its infancy, as with other personality disorders. Studies are highly exploratory and inconclusive. However, we provide a sampling of the major findings as they point toward a significant biological component underlying the development of the disorder.

Genetic Predisposition

The possibility of a genetic predisposition to BPD has been considered over the past two decades (Baron et al. 1985; Links et al. 1988; Livesley et al. 1993; Torgersen 1994, 2000; Zanarini et al. 1988). Strong evidence was established in one twin study (Torgersen et al. 2000), which found a heritability of .69 for BPD and an overall heritability of .60 for DSM-IV Cluster B personality disorders (American Psychiatric Association 1994). Genetic transmission appears to express itself through the traits of affective instability, impulsivity, self-harm, and possibly identity problems. A review of earlier family studies, but not twin studies, found minimal evidence for increased risk for BPD traits among first-degree relatives (Dahl 1994), so the genetic basis for the disorder requires continued study. However, in the case histories provided in Part II of this book, Cluster B disorders and traits are quite apparent in the patient's families, as they were in the larger sample of BPD patients studied in the Chestnut Lodge sample and in our own clinical practice.

Biological Vulnerabilities

Numerous studies suggest that BPD patients have an underlying brain dysfunction as measured by the presence of neurological soft signs, problems on intelligence tests, and difficulties in auditory-visual integration (Gardner et al. 1987; Quitkin et al. 1976). Andrulonis et al. (1980) found a wide range of problems, including episodic dyscontrol, neurological dysfunction, epilepsy, minimal brain dysfunction, and learning disabilities. Another study based on a neurobehavioral model of BPD found a predominance of learning disabilities and a trend for prematurity or low birth rate in BPD patients (Soloff and Millward 1983). Two retrospective studies of BPD patients found a significantly higher rate of unspecified "organic diagnoses" (Fyer et al. 1988; Van Reekum et al. 1993). A more recent study of BPD patients found some form of neurological vulnerability in 87.5%, with a surprisingly high occurrence of childhood speech/language disturbance, in addition to learning disabilities, ADHD, and reported complications of birth and pregnancy (Kimble et al. 1997).

A possible problem in auditory neurointegration, as measured by event-related auditory electroencephalographic potentials, also has been found (Kutcher et al. 1987). Studies using electroencephalograms (EEGs) suggest nonlocalized brain dysfunction, as evidenced by abnormal diffuse slow activity (Cowdry et al. 1985; De La Fuente et al. 1998; Snyder and Pitts 1984).

Two reports using magnetic resonance imaging (MRI) suggested abnormalities in brain structure and function in BPD patients. One study (Lyoo et al. 1998), pursuing a hypothesis regarding executive dysfunction in BPD, found a significantly smaller frontal lobe volume in BPD subjects as compared with healthy subjects. The findings regarding a smaller hippocampus in subjects with posttraumatic stress disorder (PTSD) (Stein et al. 1997) have been extended to patients with BPD. Driessen et al. (2000) found a 16% reduction in the volume of the hippocampus and an 8% smaller volume of the amygdala in a sample of 21 female BPD patients.

Another line of investigation has been to study neurobehavioral systems implicated in impulsivity and emotional dysregulation, which are core features of the disorder. Disturbances of affect and impulse regulation and self-injurious behavior are felt to be related to altered functioning of the central serotonergic system. Most studies suggest that impulse aggression is related to lower levels of serotonin (5-hydroxytryptamine; 5-HT) (Åsberg et al. 1976; Coccaro 1989; Linnoila et al. 1983).

As further support for the serotonergic hypothesis, suicide and self-injurious behaviors have been connected to lower levels of 5-HT and abnormalities in the dopaminergic system (Cheetham et al. 1988; Coccaro et al. 1989; Korpi et al. 1986; López-Ibor et al. 1990; Mann et al. 1986; Meltzer et al. 1984; Stanley et al. 2000). This response has been correlated, in at least one study, with severe and sustained traumatic stress in childhood (Rinne et al. 2000). In that study, patients who exhibited impulsive and self-injurious behavior were the victims of frequent physical and sexual abuse as children.

Using platelet measures to assess serotonergic function, Verkes et al.

(1998) found platelet 5-HT and repeated suicidal behavior were positively correlated with BPD—in particular, with chronic feelings of emptiness. The authors suggested suicidal behavior is mediated by the relationship between serotonergic function and impulsiveness as a personality trait.

There is considerable debate as to whether the neurodevelopmental problems in BPD patients are present at birth or result from child maltreatment. This chicken-and-egg controversy may never be fully resolved. However, there is a growing body of research investigating the effects of child maltreatment on brain development that may elucidate issues in this area. It appears that some temperamental structures are not functional at birth but become more complex and more organized with advancing development (Derryberry and Rothbart 1997; Rothbart and Bates 1998) and are responsive to environmental stimulation and demands. Animal model studies show that early experiences can permanently alter hormonal response to stressors (Anisman et al. 1998). The infant-maternal system of interactive caregiving is an external regulator of the infant's self-organization. The patterns of interaction are expected to modulate the infant's tendencies of arousal, attention, and reactivity to environmental stimulation (Debellis 2001).

It is thought that a significant portion of postnatal brain structuration and neural patterning occurs through the interactions of the child with the environment (Cicchetti and Tucker 1994). Early experience is also critical in determining the actualization and timing of gene expression and can make a major contribution to individual differences. Exposure to stress during early postnatal life may interact with genetic predisposition to increase the individual's susceptivity to psychopathological outcomes (Debellis et al. 1994; Meaney et al. 1996).

Cumulative stress caused by maltreatment could be manifested in dysregulation of the hypothalamic-pituitary-adrenal axis (HPA) and parasympathetic and catecholamine responses (Glaser 2000). Studies in children have shown dysregulation of the adrenal system in some of the children, but the pattern of dysfunction varies across studies (Meyer et al. 2001). In one study (Cicchetti and Rogosch 2001), the authors concluded that children with the most severe forms of maltreatment express hypercorticalism. These children experienced numerous forms of maltreatment (i.e., sexual, physical, and emotional abuse and neglect) over multiple developmental periods. It was hypothesized that this group may be at high risk for enduring neurobiological compromise. Serious cumulative maltreatment may also be a major risk factor for severe impairment and poor long-term course and outcome.

In contrast, children who are physically abused appear to express hypocorticalism (Cicchetti and Rogosch 2001). It is unclear whether this is a sign of adaptation to stress and resilience or whether it leads to stress-related disorders of bodily functioning. Hypocorticalism might also be related to an increased pain threshold and reduced perception of pain seen in BPD patients who engage in self-mutilation and other self-damaging behaviors.

In summary, biological studies of adults with BPD provide considerable support for underlying dysfunction in neurobehavioral systems. Studies of maltreated children provide indirect support that environmental factors experienced as cumulative stress and interacting with genetic factors and other vulnerabilities contribute to alterations in brain-behavior systems. We now turn to an elaboration of the environmental factors that contribute to the disorder.

ENVIRONMENTAL FACTORS

Child Maltreatment

The literature on the borderline disorder has consistently emphasized the centrality of environmental factors in the etiology of the disorder. Early theorists viewed the borderline disorder as a result of a failure to navigate successfully through the rapprochement developmental subphase related to insufficient maternal support (Masterson and Rinsley 1975; Zinner and Shapiro 1975). This view was replaced with one that hypothesized persistent parent-child failures throughout all stages of development related to unavailability or neglect (Gunderson et al. 1980), active withdrawal (Masterson and Rinsley 1975), or inconsistent support during critical developmental phases (Shapiro et al. 1975).

Child maltreatment refers to verbal, physical, and sexual abuse; emotional or physical neglect; emotional withdrawal; and inconsistent and unpredictable care. These forms of maltreatment place the individual at high risk for a variety of psychiatric disorders and maladaptive behaviors later in life (Brodsky et al. 2001; Coid et al. 2001; Gladstone et al. 1999; Kendler et al. 2000; MacMillan et al. 2001; Romans et al. 1999; Singer et al. 1989), including suicidal behaviors (Dube et al. 2001; Kaplan et al. 1995). Such forms of maltreatment have been found in a large percentage of personality disorders in general (Gibb et al. 2001; J. G. Johnson et al. 1999; Wonderlich et al. 2001), and BPD in particular (Gunderson and Sabo 1993; Herman et al. 1989; Nigg et al. 1991; Ogata et al. 1990; Paris et al. 1993; Zanarini 1997; Zanarini et al. 1989, 1997). It has been found that disturbed caregiver behavior and child maltreatment are present in early childhood, continue throughout latency and adolescence, and serve as a form of chronic stress to the developing child (Zanarini and Gunderson 1989). BPD patients are more likely than patients with other personality disorders to report having been emotionally and physically abused by a caregiver and sexually abused by a noncaregiver (Zanarini et al. 1997). The emotional abuse characteristic of early environments of BPD patients consists of failure to provide needed protection, inconsistent treatment, denial of thoughts and feelings, and placement in a parental role. Those at greatest risk for the borderline disorder have experienced biparental failure (i.e., neglect by both male and female caregivers).

It appears that children who develop borderline pathology, like adults who develop the disorder, have similar risk factors. One study (Guzder et al. 1999) found that the risk factors that differentiated the group of children with the borderline disorder from children with other psychiatric disorders were physical abuse, sexual abuse, severe neglect, and parental substance abuse or criminality. Cumulative abuse seemed to predict the disorder and was correlated with cumulative parental dysfunction.

Considerable discussion has occurred as to whether PTSD and BPD are synonymous, primarily because of the central role that trauma plays in the development of each (Gunderson and Sabo 1993; Paris 2000; Yen et al., submitted; Zlotnick et al. 2001). These disorders are frequently comorbid (McGlashan et al. 2000; Southwick et al. 1993), because they share similar symptoms (Foa et al. 1995; Marshall et al. 2001). But there are important disconfirmations (Fossati et al. 1999) and differences. Individuals with PTSD usually have specific, relatively accurate memories of the traumatic event(s), and their symptoms are triggered by exposure to a stimulus that reminds them of the event. In contrast, those with BPD have usually experienced cumulative trauma beginning at an age when such trauma is often minimized and belittled (Sjoberg and Lindbland 2002) and memory systems are insufficiently developed for the child to process and integrate the information. Early traumatic maltreatment may induce PTSD-like stress-response physiological and psychological processes or even PTSD symptoms early in childhood. However, in the course of development, the individual habituates and adapts to these experiences. They become transformed and incorporated into the personality structure and form the basis for the insecure and disorganized/disoriented attachment models described later in this chapter.

We hypothesize that BPD may, in many instances, represent developmentally "internalized" PTSD. The emotional dysregulation inherent in BPD may result, in part, from a PTSD-like generalized stress-response pattern of hyperarousal and/or numbing, but the trigger is not a specific traumatic memory. The traumatic trigger is re-created in the context of a current relationship in which closeness exposes the BPD patient to actual or feared abuse in the form of emotional neglect, abandonment, or attack. The trauma is thereby re-created and relived rather than recalled, and the psychological and physiological stress reactions are part of the person's characteristic response set within relationships and a core feature of the personality. This process will be elaborated more fully throughout this chapter.

Parental Dysfunction

Parental dysfunction, whether leading directly to child maltreatment or to milder failures in parenting, is an important etiological factor. This dysfunction includes characteristics of the parents and of the parental dyad. As illustrated in the case histories in this book, the presence, type, and severity of the parents' mental disorders influence their ability to parent and be available to the growing child. The presence of paranoid, antisocial, and narcissistic features contributes to the potential level of cruelty and violence to which the child is subject. A parent's depression may influence his or her availability and emotional responsiveness.

The quality and stability of the parents' or stepparents' relationship are also important. (The same applies for unmarried couples.) The level and kind of verbal and physical fighting and the degree of cooperation and agreement regarding parenting impact the child's development.

Adverse Life Events

Various other environmental factors, such as family illness, separation, death, availability of alternative sources of parenting, war, and poverty or extreme wealth, all impact the growing child and the caregivers' ability to parent. Perhaps equally important is the way in which the parents manage adverse life events and their ability to buffer and protect the child from being overwhelmed.

Community Support

As the case vignettes later in this book illustrate, the availability of a supportive community is an important protective factor in the course of the disorder. An extended family, which can assist the parents and provide an alternative source of encouragement and reality testing for the child, can make a difference. Similarly, a community network of church, school, and neighbors that supports the child can dilute and minimize the impact of a disturbed home environment by providing another model of how to live and interact. Similarly, the absence of these protective factors or the presence of a troubled community network could further delay and impede development.

Goodness of Fit

Another element that can play a significant etiological role is the goodness of fit between parent and child and between community and child. A child with the temperament and traits and information-processing problems described earlier could be a challenge for many parents. This type of child can also challenge a school system, church, and neighborhood. Thus, the transaction among child, caregivers, and community is a critical factor.

TEMPERAMENT, TRAITS, AND BPD

In this section, we discuss how the interaction among biological and environmental factors may express themselves through temperament, traits, and information processing.

Temperament and Traits

According to the developmental theory, the underlying genetic and neurobehavioral abnormalities described earlier interact with environmental factors and express themselves through temperament and traits. Cloninger (1998), using his seven-factor model of personality, found that BPD patients exhibit a temperament characterized by high harm avoidance (pessimism and fearfulness) and its opposite, high novelty seeking (exploration and impulsivity). These contradictory habitual responses to incoming emotional stimuli create an inherent conflict in novel situations. In this model, BPD patients also exhibit low reward dependence, which refers to a lack of facility in the development of conditioned signals to reward, especially to social cues. This factor is hypothesized to result in a detached and insensitive response to social communication. Such response, in turn, could interfere with the development of a secure attachment, especially under conditions of child maltreatment.

Similar contradictory personality traits are found using the five-factor model of personality (Digman 1990; McCrae and John 1992). BPD patients score high on neuroticism (emotional instability, worry, shyness) and its opposite, extraversion (gregariousness, assertiveness, and excitement seeking). They score low on straightforwardness and compliance in interpersonal relationships, which could parallel the insensitive responsiveness to social cues found in Cloninger's model. Finally, BPD patients also score low on achievement striving (Widiger et al. 1994). These factor-analytic findings provide indirect support for the presence of affective instability as an underlying temperament or trait, as it is similar to the characteristics of harm avoidance and neuroticism. Impulsivity also is suggested, as it is a maladaptive expression of novelty seeking and extraversion.

Information-Processing Deficits

Abnormalities in brain structure and function and temperamental deviations amplified by cumulative stress can contribute to information-processing and integrative deficits. A number of empirical studies have found a high prevalence of cognitive disturbances in BPD patients that appear stable over time (Chopra and Beatson 1986; George and Soloff 1986; Gunderson 1984; O'Connell et al. 1989; Pope et al. 1985; Silk et al. 1989; Sternbach et al. 1992). These disturbances have been characterized as odd reasoning (superstitiousness, magical thinking, a sixth sense, clairvoyance, telepathy), dichotomous (black-white) thinking, overvalued ideas, unusual perceptions, severe dissociation, paranoia, and transient psychotic thought (Zanarini et al. 1990). These disturbances seem to occur as frequently as they do in patients with schizotypal personality disorder (Sternbach et al. 1992) and are a stable part of BPD.

Many early studies using psychological tests provide evidence for cognitive dysfunction. Studies that have examined the Rorschach protocols of BPD patients (Berg 1983; M. T. Singer 1977; M. T. Singer and Larson 1981; Sugarman 1980) found deviant thought and communication patterns, an inability to maintain or shift cognitive set, and odd reasoning. Exner (1986) described the BPD cognitive style on the Rorschach as underincorporative and indicative of an "immature and or inadequate organizational structure" (p. 469). BPD patients also appear unable to reflect on their performance on the Rorschach and cannot detect errors in reasoning (Berg 1983).

It had been thought that patients with the borderline disorder performed normally on structured tests such as the Wechsler Adult Intelligence Scale (WAIS; Wechsler 1958, 1981) but that their cognitive ability regressed on unstructured tasks such as the Rorschach. However, closer examination of WAIS protocols found greater intra- and intertest scatter, odd word usage, disruptions of boundaries between concepts, and lapses in logical thinking on tasks requiring extensive use of language for these patients (Berg 1983; Carr et al. 1979; Widiger 1982). On the Minnesota Multiphasic Personality Inventory (MMPI), BPD patients have consistent elevation on the F scale, which indicates odd and unusual thinking, and a peak on scale 8, which is indicative of a thought disorder (Patrick 1984). They also characteristically have a "floating profile"

(Newmark and Sines 1972), which includes elevation on many clinical scales and is indicative of an inability to discriminate among emotional states.

These earlier findings were confirmed through a series of neuropsychological studies that compared BPD patients with control subjects (Carpenter et al. 1993; Judd and Ruff 1993; O'Leary et al. 1991; Swirsky-Sacchetti et al. 1993). These studies consistently found deficits in visuospatial learning, memory and fluency, and verbal learning of complex novel verbal information in the BPD patients compared with the control subjects. The findings were consistent after control for medications, current major depression, substance abuse histories, and psychiatric settings. On the basis of these studies, as well as Luria's (1973) theory of brain functioning, it has been hypothesized that these problems represent a dysfunction in BPD patients' ability to convert concrete perceptions into functional patterns and to integrate and transform complex information into symbolic schemas in a rapid and fluid manner (Judd and Ruff 1993).

Pine (1986) proposed that the borderline disorder in children emerged as a result of an interaction between constitutional neuropsychological defects and early trauma. As a result, children with the borderline disorder felt overwhelmed by environmental stimuli and exhibited problems in learning, social interaction, and coping ability. Supporting his view, one neuropsychological study of children found problems in planning and cognitive fluency and flexibility, independent of comorbidity with conduct disorder and attention-deficit disorder (Paris et al. 1999). These children exhibited more difficulty completing tasks, made more errors, failed to learn from errors, and appeared unable to achieve an overall conceptualization of the tasks set by the test. Another study (Lincoln et al. 1998) found that the patterns of evoked response potentials in children with the borderline disorder, an indirect measure of information-processing ability, were qualitatively different from those in comparison groups. Further, these children had impairments in their executive control, motor planning, and reaction speed and in their ability to discriminate and replicate auditory information.

We suspect that these information-processing problems play a unique role in the development of the disorder. We hypothesize that these deficits interfere with the processing of contradictory emotional, sensory, and motor signals; the translation of nonverbal information into verbal codes; and/or meaningful discrimination and prioritization of divergent visual and verbal interpersonal responses that are characteristic of maltreating environments. These abilities are central to the development of abstract representational schemes of interpersonal relationships.

These problems may also be expressed as a form of learning disability that interferes with interpersonal learning. Palombo (1995) discussed how children with nonverbal learning disabilities decode social situations and emotional situations in idiosyncratic ways. Lai (1990) proposed that the right hemisphere, which is involved in intermodal integration and the processing and modulating of emotions, may be implicated in the development of social skills. The findings on MRI and positron emission tomography (PET) scans, which suggest that BPD patients may have a brain dysfunction in the amygdala and hippocampus (areas critical to the processing of emotional information), lend support to our hypothesis.

Dissociation

We propose that that the information-processing and integrative problems described earlier in this chapter are manifested through the clinical phenomena of dissociation. Dissociation has been traditionally understood as a defensive coping strategy that protects one from the overwhelming emotion and intolerable information induced by traumatic events. Dissociation may, however, be related to an interaction between failed information processing and automatic defensive processes (Linotti 1999). The clinical description of dissociation refers to disruptions in the normal integration of memories, perception, and identity associated with trauma (American Psychiatric Association 1994). Dissociation can also be understood as a failure of information processing (Bower and Sivers 1998), possibly related to release of large quantities of stress hormones and neurotransmitters during traumatic or highly emotionally arousing situations. This would lead to high levels of activation of the sympathetic nervous system that could interfere with the processing of information. It would be greatly amplified in those with a preexisting processing problem.

BPD patients experience a moderate to severe level and a wide variety of dissociative experiences, including absorption, amnesia, and depersonalization (Zanarini et al. 2000). Although dissociation is commonly viewed as occurring along a continuum from normal to psychopathological, it has been proposed that this conceptualization be replaced with Janet's view on dissociation as a rare discontinuity in and extreme deviation from consciousness (Waller et al. 1996). From this standpoint, dissociation is a completely separate construct that is inherently psychopathological.

Although some studies have found associations between clinically significant levels of dissociation and childhood trauma (Macfie et al. 2001; Putnam 1993; Strick and Wilcox 1991; Waldinger et al. 1994), other studies provide support for the hypothesis that dissociation is related to biological rather than environmental factors. These studies explored the presence of dissociation in patients with and without histories of trauma and concluded that dissociation refers to a form of psychopathology that is not necessarily connected to trauma (Bremner and Brett 1997; Waller et al. 1996; Zweig-Frank et al. 1994a, 1994b). This possibility has been further supported in a longitudinal study of high-risk children who develop dissociation (Ogawa et al. 1997).

The brain-behavior basis for dissociation has been proposed as lying between a primitive subcortical emotional conditioning system and a cortically based cognitive system that mediates conscious awareness of threatening stimuli and ability to talk about them (i.e., become conscious of them) (Bower and Sivers 1998). Learning about emotional scenes involves adrenocortical hormones and the amygdala complex (Cahill et al. 1996). In studies of individuals with PTSD, it has been proposed that the hippocampus appears to act as a critical structure for bringing together and binding a variety of inputs to those multiple neocortical regions that are encoding and recording the various parts of a traumatic experience (McClelland et al. 1995). Abnormalities of hippocampal functioning may affect the binding and integration function, and sensory parts of an episode may be stored in isolation from an association to the cortically based experiencing ego or self (Bower and Sivers 1998; Bremner et al. 1995; Krystal et al. 1995). As evidenced by the findings on structural abnormalities in the amygdala and hippocampus described earlier, this area may be the site of the information-processing problems in BPD patients.

In a longitudinal study of dissociation in children, child's IQ, as measured by the Wechsler Preschool and Primary Scale of Intelligence (WPPSI), was found to predict dissociative behavior from toddlerhood to grade school (Ogawa et al. 1997). Because the WPPSI also measures various forms of information processing, this finding also supports the presence of cognitive problems as possibly underlying psychopathological dissociation. Another relevant finding from this study is that children classified as having disorganized attachments, which, as described later in this chapter, is a central feature of the disorder, were likely to have high dissociation scores in adolescence and young adulthood. Because the predictors of dissociation in young adulthood were all measured in the child's first 2 years of life, this finding serves as a powerful possible validation that information-processing deficits are present early and are influencing the course of attachment. This finding also supports the importance of early experience for later development and the strength of the developmental pathway model.

THE ATTACHMENT SYSTEM

We hypothesize that the central pathway for the development of the disorder is through the attachment system. Vygotsky's theory on the development of higher mental functions (Rieber and Carton 1987) provides a useful bridge between biological and environmental theories of etiology. Vygotsky posited that the higher functions of the brain develop during the period of communication between the child and adult, when function was shared between two people. The child begins to apply to himself or herself the same forms of behavior that were applied to him or her by others, and inner speech, the voice of and dialogue with the parent, develops. These transactions eventually become encoded in memory and form abstract representations of relationships that guide and regulate behavior. Over the course of early development, these patterns form a model of attachment regarding how to get one's needs for security and a safety met. The relationship between parent and child is where biology becomes biography. The relationship between treatment team members and patient is where both biology and biography can be modified or ameliorated.

Attachment is defined as a behavioral control system that maintains the infant's safety and survival through access to parental protection, care, and nurture (Bowlby 1969/1982, 1973, 1980). This system, which is similar to that found in nonhuman primates, functions to regulate infant safety as it did in the environments in which it originally evolved. The attachment behavioral system is activated by stress and has as its goal the reduction of arousal and restoration of a sense of security. As such, affect regulation becomes a primary goal of the attachment system.

Attachment theory posits that when the child feels consistently and sensitively cared for, a secure relationship is established (Bowlby 1969/1982). Attachment is genetically programmed in all mammals as a necessary condition for survival and appears in humans across cultures by the age of 7 months. Within the matrix of a secure attachment, the child is able to maintain flexible attention so that she or he can explore the world and master developmental tasks, including emotional and behavioral regulation, coherent sense of self in relation to others, and personal identity.

Infant-mother relationships develop in a reciprocal bidirectional manner (Sameroff and Fiese 1990, 2000). Infant characteristics play a role in the formation of attachment relationships (Goldsmith and Alansky 1987) in that their temperament and traits influence how the caregiver will respond. However, some evidence suggests that in clinical samples with depressed and maltreating mothers, the mother appears to play a more important role than the child in shaping the quality of the attachment relationship (van IJzendoorn et al. 1992). In those who develop BPD, we suspect that the child is in greater need of adequate parenting because of her or his greater biological vulnerability. Thus, maltreatment may extract a higher cost than it does in more resilient children, and in this sense the parents may play a more important role in the genesis of the disorder.

We hypothesize that the formation of a secure organized attachment system did not occur in the child who develops BPD. Instead, the child develops an insecure and disorganized attachment system that contains multiple loosely integrated modes of relating characterized as preoccupied (anxious and ambivalent) and/or dismissing–detached. These multiple modes refer to different cognitive schemas or abstract representations of attachment that are organized to meet needs for safety, security, and self-worth. We further propose that the variations in course and severity of the disorder are related to 1) the degree of disorganization of the attachment system that refers to the lack of elaboration and integration of abstract representations and 2) the predominant attachment model that has developed: preoccupied or dismissing. Treatment works toward stabilizing and integrating the attachment system into a more organized preoccupied and/or dismissing mode.

The state of mind regarding attachment that develops in infancy and early childhood is carried forward into all subsequent close relationships through the construction of abstract symbolic representational models (Cassidy 1990; Cicchetti and Schneider-Rosen 1986; Sroufe and Fleeson 1988). These models are the result of repeated interpersonal interactions that have been encoded in memory as prototypic (Stern 1985). During optimal development, when a secure attachment pattern is formed, the cumulative experience with varied caregivers is encoded in memory in an integrated manner and forms a working model that allows for the cognitive generation of novel responses to new interpersonal situations (Crittenden 1990) and serves as a reliable method for reducing anxiety and regulating negative emotion. It enables the child, and later the adult, to respond with flexible attention to environmental demands.

In contrast, the individual who develops BPD has been unable to integrate various models of relating into one that is prototypical. Instead, she or he is forced to rely on multiple models that leave her or him vulnerable to being continuously overwhelmed with affect and subject to behavioral disorganization. This, in turn, interferes with all aspects of development.

To elaborate on this further, we provide a brief description of how attachment status is classified in infants and adults. Over the past 25 years, the work of Bowlby (1969/1982, 1973, 1980) has been extended to the development of classification systems for infant, toddler, and adult attachment patterns. Numerous studies have been conducted on low-risk samples of infants and mothers to determine attachment patterns in nonclinical populations across varying cultures, and more recently these classification systems have been applied to clinical populations (Hesse 1999).

Infant/Toddler Attachment Classification

Infant attachment classifications were derived through studies based on the Ainsworth Strange Situation procedure (Ainsworth et al. 1978)—a research method based on observations of how infants and toddlers react to separation from their mother. These classifications refer to the child's characteristic method or modus operandi for maintaining proximity to the mother so as to obtain comfort and care and regulate affect. The child's attachment pattern is described as 1) organized/secure; 2) organized/insecure; 3) insecure, with either an avoidant or resistant/ambivalent pattern; or 4) disorganized/disoriented (Ainsworth and Wittig 1969; Ainsworth et al. 1978; Main 2000; Main and Solomon 1990).

Securely attached children have highly organized and predictable approaches for maintaining proximity to the mother. They show signs of missing her on first separation, and they cry during the second separation. As soon as mother returns, they reach for her actively and after brief contact are able to return to play. Secure children are hypothesized to have been sensitively and reliably responded to when distressed. They have learned that mother will be prompt and comforting in response to distress and can relax and divert their attention to the larger world once she is present.

Children with an insecure avoidant attatchment pattern also have a highly organized approach to maintaining proximity. They maintain a focus on the toys in the room. They do not cry on separation and appear overly involved in play as mother leaves and returns to the room. They act as if they are not attached and it does not matter whether mother is present or not. They maintain behavioral organization by diverting their attention away from mother, ignoring her as she enters the room and leaning away when picked up. These mothers have responded to their child's expression of need with consistent rejecting behaviors such as ignoring or pushing away. The child learns that the best way to maintain mother's involvement is through dismissing her apparent importance and acting as if she were not needed. Despite her or his apparent disregard of the mother, the child experiences considerable physiological distress as mother leaves and returns (Spangler and Grossmann 1993).

Children with an insecure resistant/ambivalent attachment pattern are preoccupied with the parent throughout the procedure. Their attention is fixed on the mother. This approach, like the insecure avoidant attachment approach, is organized and predictable, although the intense affect makes it appear more disorganized. When mother returns to the room, the child may seem angry and alternately seek and resist the parent's attempts to comfort. The child is unable to settle down and return to play. The child appears to maintain behavioral organization through a hyperfocus on the parent to the exclusion of exploration of the room and toys. This pattern develops in response to maternal insensitivity, and specifically with unpredictable responsiveness. We speculate that over time the child learns that the most effective method for obtaining and maintaining parental care is through displays of continuous distress. However, this method diverts the child away from other important developmental tasks.

Children with a disorganized or disoriented pattern, which we propose is characteristic of BPD patients, display a diverse array of odd, disorganized, disoriented, or overtly conflicted behaviors during the infant Strange Situation (Hesse and Main 2000). Their attention collapses under the stress of parental separation and reunion. The child can neither avoid nor ignore the stress caused by the parental behaviors, nor can he or she develop a strategy to maintain behavioral organization (M. Main, R. Goldwyn, "Adult Attachment Scoring and Classification Systems," ms. in preparation). Disorganized attachment occurs in some children with neurological impairment and may appear in conjunction with extended periods of isolation (Hesse and Main 2000). In maltreatment samples, 48%–80% of the children have been classified as having a disorganized attachment classification (Carlson et al, 1989; Lyons-Ruth and Block 1996; van IJzendoorn 1995). We speculate that these odd and disoriented behaviors represent both behavioral disorganization and rudimentary attachment patterns that cannot cohere into an organized pattern. We imagine that this disorganized and random responding is the early indication of dissociation and of the child's inability to interpret and integrate divergent emotional and sensorimotor information into coherent patterns.

A key feature that is hypothesized to underlie the development of unresolved/disorganized/disoriented attachment patterns is frightening behavior on the part of the caregiver (Hesse and Main 2000; Main and Hesse 1990). Fear initiates a fight-or-flight response, but when this response is blocked, disorganization can result. When the child is distressed, the parent, who may feel angry, overwhelmed, and frightened herself and unable to understand what the child needs, responds with behaviors that may frighten the child. These behaviors can include a disoriented or frightened face, withdrawal, silence or yelling, hitting, criticism, and/or invalidating comments that heighten rather then reduce the child's fear and anxiety. These kinds of behaviors may also be experienced as an absence of care or neglect, which is experienced as abandonment. Bowlby (1973) suggested that "[c]hildren lacking confidence in the availability of care as a result would be prone to intense or chronic fear" (p. 202).

The frightening behavior of the caregiver creates an inherent paradox for the child. The place or haven of safety to which the child is biologically programmed and compelled to return is simultaneously that which frightens and raises the child's anxiety to intolerable levels. However, this paradoxical relationship becomes embedded in memory in separate schemas, one being the safe relationship and the other the frightening and maltreating relationship. This helps to explain why BPD patients repeatedly return to abusive or maltreating relationships; these relationships represent a place of safety in the mind.

A growing body of child literature provides support for the later expression of disorganized attachment in infancy as the borderline disorder. At age 6 years, children who were classified as having had a disorganized attachment pattern as an infant exhibit role-inverting behavior—either controlling and punitive or excessively and inappropriately solicitous (van IJzendoorn et al. 1999). This behavior is very typical in borderline children and adults. Disruptive and aggressive behavior in middle childhood has been linked to early disorganization with the mother (Lyons-Ruth and Block 1996; van IJzendoorn et al. 1999). Again, these behavior patterns are characteristic of BPD patients. Finally, disorganized behavior in infancy has also been found to be predictive of dissociative behavior and experiences from middle childhood to 17 years of age (Carlson 1998), another feature of the disorder.

Adult Attachment Classification

A classification system similar to that developed for children has been developed for adults using the Berkeley Adult Attachment Interview (AAI; George et al. 1984, 1985, 1996; M. Main, R. Goldwyn, "Adult Attachment Scoring and Classification Systems," ms. in preparation). The adult classification system also articulates secure, avoidant or dismissing, preoccupied (ambivalent/resistant), and disorganized patterns but adds a "cannot classify" category. This system was based on an implicit understanding that early nonverbal, behaviorally enacted attachment patterns observed in the Strange Situation procedure are transformed into complex representational processes embedded in memory. These processes are manifested through the way in which an individual describes her or his relationships and life history to an interviewer.

The AAI, similar in some respects to an initial clinical interview, assesses the organization and coherence of the person's narrative and her or his ability to stay focused on the collaborative task at hand. An important aspect of this assessment is the person's ability to integrate the emotion generated by the interview into the historical narrative. The patient's ability to maintain attentional flexibility and self-monitoring during the interview, as expressed through the coherence, quality, and relevance of her or his language, provides a window into her or his mode of relating (Hesse 1999).

This body of attachment research provides growing empirical support for the long-held clinical belief that parent-child relationships play a central role in the transmission of representational models of self and others. A correlation between infant and adult classifications has been found and has been replicated in more than 18 samples (Hesse 1999). It has been validated that a parent's state of mind with respect to attachment as measured by the AAI is predictive of the infant's attachment classification on the Strange Situation procedure (Main et al. 1985; van IJzendoorn 1995). This finding suggests that representational processes or interpersonal schemas of the parent are likely mediators of differences in parental caregiving behavior (Main 2000). Similarly, it was determined that attachment patterns in low-risk samples appear to be relatively stable across at least three generations (Benoit and Parker 1994), and a simple parent-child transmission model was found to account for the results. The cumulative research findings support the validity and reliability of both infant and adult classifications and provide evidence that attachment models are relatively stable over time. These findings lend further support to the central role of attachment in the development of BPD.

The relevance and application of attachment theory and research to a study of BPD has just begun. Gunderson (1996) has applied attachment theory to an understanding of the BPD patient's difficulty in being alone and the need for therapist availability. Fonagy et al. (2000) have proposed that BPD patients may have a disorganized attachment related to their frightening experiences with caregivers and that this interferes with the development of reflective function, which helps to integrate self-other representations. Two preliminary studies (Fonagy et al. 1996; Patrick et al. 1994) that used the AAI to study BPD patients found that

BPD patients had a preoccupied and disorganized/unresolved state of mind regarding attachment. Descriptions of frightening events repeatedly and inappropriately interrupted responses to a variety of queries, and the patients were found to have representations or schemas about early attachments that were preoccupied, confused, and fearful. A study that is currently under way is exploring changes in attachment classifications of BPD patients as part of a larger study of the effectiveness of manualized Transference Focused Psychotherapy (Clarkin et al. 2001).

MULTIPLE MODELS

We hypothesize that BPD patients are unable to develop a secure fully organized integrated attachment model related to the severity of and interaction among their neurodevelopmental vulnerabilities and environmental factors. Instead, they develop a predominately insecure, disorganized, and poorly integrated model that fluctuates among features of the preoccupied (anxious and ambivalent) and dismissing/detached modes. Under person-specific stressful conditions, the patient's predominant model collapses, with attendant emotional, behavioral, and cognitive disorganization and dysregulation.

These multiple models underlie the emotional, behavioral, and cognitive dysregulation, the stably unstable interpersonal relationships, and the identity confusion so characteristic of the disorder and interfere with the development of sustained intimate relationships. We propose that the predominant mode of insecure attachment (preoccupied or dismissing) and the degree of disorganization under stressful conditions constitute the primary determinant of variations in BPD course and severity of impairment. The possibility for increased organization of the attachment system also explains the significant potential for improvement in many BPD patients.

Bowlby (1973) first elaborated the construct of "multiple working models" to explain why some patients show disorganized thinking regarding their attachment relationships. He speculated that their working models were contradictory or incompatible. Main (1991) has posited that multiple models are linked to poorly developed metacognitive functioning related to the child's being forced to encode experiences that are highly contradictory.

How might multiple models develop? Attachment patterns are initially developed as sensorimotor schemas that appear prior to the emergence of language (Lane and Schwartz 1987; Stern 1985). These schemas include elaborate memories that combine sensation, perception, action, emotion, and goals that occur in temporal, physical, and causal relations. These schemas evolve through complex interactions between the child and caregivers mediated by touch, smell, affective expressions, nonverbal gestures, and speech. They reflect the quality and kind of care received.

The schemas become increasingly detailed and complex as caregivers and child interact around the following developmental needs: 1) regulation of arousal and emotional intensity through calming and soothing behaviors; 2) regulation of emotional intensity through correctly identifying the child's intentions and needs and labeling feelings; 3) regulation of the child's curiosity and engagement with the world by providing needed structure and safety while offering opportunities and encouragement for exploration; and 4) regulation of somatic states through provision of healthy diet, regular meals, proper care when ill, and transitions from wakeful fatigue to sleep (Stern 1985). The transactions that occur are encoded in memory, and the child gradually learns to apply to herself or himself and enact with others the quality and kind of care that was provided in the manner in which it was learned.

LANGUAGE AND THE GOAL-CORRECTED PARTNERSHIP

In normal development, sensorimotor schemas become increasingly symbolic, abstract, and integrated through the evolving linguistic dialogue between parent and child. Vygotsky noted that speech gives the child the power to free herself or himself from and go beyond the limits of immediate impressions (Rieber and Carton 1987). As such, language serves as the primary medium for integration and order in human mental life. As the child develops language and engages in verbal dialogue with caregivers, emotions become increasingly complex and differentiated and are linked in various assemblies to cognitions. Language—and more importantly the dialogue between parents and child—fosters cognitive development, a sense of self, and integrated representations of self and other.

Between the ages of 2 and 5, parent and child engage in rudimentary verbal discussions of feelings and plans that Bowlby (1969/1982) termed a "goal-corrected partnership." Through these transactions children learn to use language to communicate and gain skill in conducting a reciprocal relationship. As part of this process, they develop pragmatic language, which refers to discourse skills and words and phrases that initiate and sustain conversation. Words as symbols gradually replace sensorimotor schemas with abstract representations.

Through verbal discussion the child's anxiety is reduced, and she or he feels increased mastery over intense emotional states. The secure child learns that emotional expression will not overwhelm the parent and that emotion is tolerable and shareable (Malatesta-Magai 1991). This fosters social skills and the child's capacity to learn how to cope with emotionally arousing situations.

In maltreated children, language is impoverished in productivity, complexity, and content, but especially in use of pragmatic language (i.e., questions, descriptive utterances, discourse skills) (Coster et al. 1989). Receptive language appears intact, but expressive language is affected (Beeghly and Cicchetti 1994). In particular, maltreated children produce fewer words referring to their internal state. This leads to fewer dyadic exchanges about feeling states and an impoverished, disorganized emotional vocabulary, which are hypothesized to interfere further with the acquisition of interpersonal regulatory skills and increasing self-other differentiation (Beeghly and Cicchetti 1994).

We assume that for those who develop the borderline disorder, a goal-corrected partnership is never formed or is repeatedly derailed by maltreatment and adverse life events. Parents may communicate through contradictory and confused verbal and nonverbal messages. Content, vocal tone, emotion, and facial gesture are incongruous with intentions. Verbal dialogue does not serve its function to clarify, symbolize, and regulate, but instead obfuscates, frustrates, and frightens. The child is unable to learn how, when, and under what circumstances to use language to get needs met with appropriate subtlety. The child who goes on to develop BPD, related to her or his information-processing problems, is especially dependent on the parent to translate the interpersonal world and learn effective communication. Without this assistance, she or he has no choice but to speak through behavioral action patterns. In this sense, the BPD patient is a speechless child. She or he has not learned to use language in pragmatic meaningful ways to engage others, to express self, or to assert need.

COGNITIVE DYSFUNCTION

We have described the BPD patient's problems with information processing and integration of interpersonal information and how these contribute to dissociation and multiple models. We now further elaborate how cognitive development in the interpersonal arena goes awry.

Metacognitive Monitoring

The cumulative effect of these problems is an impaired capacity for metacognitive monitoring in the interpersonal arena, also referred to as *reflective function. Metacognitive monitoring* (Flavell 1979) refers to the ability to observe oneself while speaking and to detect errors in reasoning or inconsistencies in one's narrative—to think about thinking. *Metacognitive knowledge* refers to the recognition of an appearance-reality distinction that things may not be as they appear and that appearances are never certain (Flavell et al. 1983). It also refers to an awareness that the same things might appear differently to different persons and that our thoughts vary from day to day about the same topic (Forguson and Gopnik 1988). This knowledge requires a high degree of analytic, synthetic, and flexible thinking and appears related to secure attachment and an integrated representational model (Main 2000). Metacognition corresponds to the level of formal operations in Piaget's theory, and empathy is the hallmark of formal operations in the interpersonal arena (Lane and Schwartz 1987). Metacognition and empathy are impaired in individuals with BPD, and the extent to which these individuals are capable of developing this ability will determine their long-term course and outcome.

Denial, Splitting, and Projection

Without metacognition, BPD individuals must rely on the simpler cognitive processes of denial, splitting, and projection to analyze interpersonal situations. These mental processes, applied to BPD and elaborated by Kernberg (1967, 1975), are usually understood as defenses against painful emotion but are here understood as immature cognitive processes and signs of lack of integration and dissociation.

Denial is a manifestation of dissociation during painful events and the absence of cognitive processing of these events as part of one's interpersonal schema. It represents a lack of integration of the emotional impact and consequences of significant events on the individual. For example, many BPD patients initially "deny" early maltreatment because they have not processed and integrated the emotional experience with its interpersonal meaning. Similarly, a woman who has been beaten by her husband will "deny" the pain and interpersonal meaning. She has not integrated the emotional and practical import of her husband's actions with her schema of him as the "man she loves."

Splitting is an inability to think dichotomously—that is, to entertain opposing thoughts and understand that others have competing motivations and separate states of mind. Significant others are experienced as all good or bad and subsequently idealized or devalued. Kernberg (1967) noted that "[s]plitting interferes with the ability to synthesize which normally brings about . . . abstraction and integration of an object relationship" (p. 672).

Projection refers to the attribution of one's own thoughts and emotions, usually negative ones, to another. This process reflects a lack of awareness of and inability to identify oneself as the owner of certain emotions. Projection incorporates elements of denial and splitting and contributes to a variety of cognitive distortions, paranoia, and paranoid states.

Stress-Related Paranoid and Other Psychotic States

Related to the cognitive problems just described, BPD patients are vulnerable to a disorganization of cognitive processing in the form of brief, acute paranoid and other psychotic states and a more generalized inability to problem solve. This usually occurs when attachment to significant others is seriously threatened through abandonment or attack. These states represent a breakdown in the processing of information and in the patient's attempt to restore meaning. In a paranoid state, the BPD patient can become convinced that a significant other is out to harm her or him and will mobilize action to protect the self. Around loss or abandonment or in the midst of a major depression, the BPD patient may hear voices of a loved one or experience other psychotic-like phenomena.

EMOTIONAL AND BEHAVIORAL DYSREGULATION AND DYSFUNCTION

Emotional Dysregulation

Delayed or distorted emotional development, or emotional dysregulation, is a further developmental outcome and core feature of BPD. Linehan (1995) has proposed that emotional dysregulation is the core problem for BPD patients and that its impact extends beyond the sphere of affect to permeate all aspects of the individual's life. Although we do not think it is the core problem, but rather another aspect of their complex developmental disorder, we do believe that it permeates all aspects of the patient's life because of the central importance of emotion to human adaptation. As with cognitive development, BPD patients move between a sensorimotor and preoperational stage of emotional development. Characteristic of this stage of development, affect is primarily experienced as a bodily sensation and an action tendency based on undifferentiated states of pleasure and displeasure or an awareness of individual feelings that have an either-or quality (Lane and Schwartz 1987).

BPD patients have not fully developed the ability either to differentiate emotions or to experience multiple emotions as part of a single emotional reaction. The awareness that one can feel a blend of emotions that might be contradictory is missing. Related to this, BPD patients recover slowly from an aroused emotional state, as do young children. Further, they are unable to connect emotional states to an interpersonal precipitant except globally. Their language consists primarily of basic emotional state words such as "feel bad." They face adult situations with a child's emotional repertoire.

Ribot (see Rieber and Carton 1987, p. 326) commented that the emotions, like "a state within a state," are the sole domain of the human mind that can only be understood retrospectively. Emotions are reflexive and preverbal. From an evolutionary perspective, they are part of the bioregulatory system for survival and signal the organism when to fight or flee and regulate our internal state so as to maintain homeostasis. A central function of emotion is to signal danger or threat to the organism. It automatically provides us with a signal for survival-oriented behaviors.

Emotions are also a fundamental stepping-stone for the process of planning specific and novel forms of adaptive responses (Damasio 1999). Our ability to discern fine shades of emotion contributes to our greater adaptive capacity. The better able we are to read others' emotional cues, the more effective we can be socially. As described earlier, the development of a language of emotion assists in its modulation.

All aspects of BPD patients' emotional development are adversely impacted. Their emotional dysregulation is an expression of their emotional vulnerability and their inability to modulate emotional responses (e.g., Gunderson and Zanarini 1989; Linehan 1993, 1995; Links et al. 2000; Parker et al. 2000; Sanislow et al. 2002). However, a difficulty with identification of emotional states and their precipitants is an important contributor to their vulnerability and poor capacity for modulation. BPD patients frequently misread interpersonal situations and overreact or underreact, depending on this misinterpretation. If we liken modulation to the regulation of a gas stove, BPD patients turn the heat up either too high or not high enough; they cannot turn the heat down or turn it off prematurely. These swings from hyperarousal to underarousal are related to a misinterpretation of emotional signals, which in turn interferes with planning adaptive responses.

Emotional dysregulation is typically expressed through affective instability, periodic states of "emptiness," emotional numbing, aversive tension, and intense anger. Affective instability, a key aspect of emotional dysregulation, is related to the BPD patient's emotional vulnerability, which is characterized by an unusual sensitivity to personally significant emotional stimuli (low threshold) coupled with abnormally strong reactions to those stimuli. Once elicited, these emotional responses are slower than normal to return to baseline. As Linehan (1995) notes, "[T]hese individuals are easily provoked and their emotional responses are extreme and long-lasting" (p. 11). When not affected personally, BPD patients often appear impervious to emotion. At other times, they report feeling numb to what the therapist would expect to be a highly arousing emotional experience.

It is difficult to describe "emptiness," but we liken it to a feeling of the presence of absence. It is accompanied by an awareness that something is missing. We speculate at these times the BPD patient feels disconnected from significant others and that this state is experienced as numbness. Without connection and the attendant motivating emotions, the BPD patient (and perhaps all humans) cannot determine a course of action. This is a potentially dangerous state from an evolutionary survival point of view. When it persists, the patient becomes increasingly dysphoric. The dysphoria can trigger a variety of potentially self-damaging behaviors that represent an attempt to dispel it and restore more normal feeling states.

BPD patients also have particular difficulty with the modulation of anger. Anger functions to alert us to frustrating events or obstacles blocking goal-oriented behavior. Anger also triggers assertive thought and energizes action to ameliorate frustration (Cicchetti et al. 1995). Borderline patients experienced enormous frustration of need and helplessness throughout childhood. Their poor emotional vocabulary further contributes to high levels of inarticulate frustration. This frustration, in combination with their underlying contradictory temperamental dispositions, creates a substrate of dysphoria and disgruntlement that can easily turn into anger when fueled by cognitive distortions and misinterpretations of interpersonal situations.

As a result, anger has developed as an "umbrella" affect state for BPD patients, within which are embedded frustration, hurt, disappointment, sadness, and revenge. Because anger contains so many affects, it is a frequent response to many interpersonal situations and can erupt into rage, with potentially dangerous and destructive interpersonal consequences.

Finally, most individuals with BPD develop Axis I depressive and anxiety disorders. These episodes can be acute, as in a major depressive episode and panic attack, or chronic, as in generalized anxiety and dysthymia. Chronic stress, affective instability, and dysphoria contribute to these Axis I conditions.

Behavioral Dysregulation

Behavioral dysregulation is another core dimension and is related to inadequate emotional development. Because they have not accurately interpreted emotional signals and are unable to modulate their reactions, BPD patients are hindered in their planning of adaptive and goal-oriented responses. Consequently, they tend to overreact or underreact behaviorally on the basis of the emotional information they have received. Their behaviors mirror their affects and range from appropriate to dysregulated to disorganized.

BPD patients reenact instead of remember early transactions with parents that were traumatic. Thus, emotions trigger action patterns that are often dramatic and provocative because of their deep interpersonal meaning. When overwhelmed with affect, the BPD patient can react in a highly impulsive manner through reckless behaviors that endanger self or others and through suicidal or homicidal behaviors. Other intense affect states prompt impulsive and/or compulsive reliance on pleasurable activities such as eating, sex, buying, and using drugs and alcohol. These behaviors are a means to modulate intense affect; avoid feelings of dysphoria, loneliness, and abandonment; and dispel emptiness and numbness, but they usually become self-damaging.

Intense emotional states, which often combine multiple affects (i.e., sadness, fear, anger, revenge, and longing), also contribute to suicidal and self-mutilating behaviors. BPD patients' experience of anger results in its frequent behavioral expression through tirades, suicidal or self-mutilating behaviors, antisocial acts, lawsuits, and work grievances. Under extreme stress, their behavioral strategies collapse, and the patients can become highly disorganized and random. One patient wandered the streets in a state of panic, calling her case manager from telephone booths throughout the city, threatening suicide. Eventually the police sent a helicopter unit to find her.

Factor analysis supports behavioral dysregulation as a core feature of BPD (Sanislow et al. 2000, 2002). It appears to be heritable (Coccaro et al. 1993) and stable over years (Links et al. 2000), and its constellation of behaviors appears to be associated biologically with the brain's serotonergic system, as noted earlier (Coccaro et al. 1989; Siever and Trestman 1993). The traits of extraversion and novelty seeking that were identified as underlying the disorder may also make up part of

its heritability. This factor is shared by other Cluster B personality disorders (i.e., narcissistic, antisocial, histrionic) and is expressed differently by sex. Males are more substance-abusing and antisocial; females
are more likely to have eating disorders or to engage in self-destructive
behaviors (D. M. Johnson et al., submitted; Soloff et al. 2000). These sex
differences characterize the non-BPD general population as well, suggesting that the distinctions are related not uniquely to the borderline
disorder but to cultural norms.

Developmental Pathway for Emotional and Behavioral Dysfunction

As elaborated above, emotions are designed from an evolutionary and
developmental perspective to organize and motivate behavior. Basic
emotional responses and expressions, such as interest, joy, sadness, anger, and fear, appear during infancy before the development of thought
and language. They appear to be preadapted to the environment and require no cognitive construction for activation or expression (Izard 1989).

Emotions are expressed through a variety of behaviors, so that emotion and behavior are inextricably bound together throughout the
course of development. Emotion, as expressed through behaviors, signals the infant's inner state and serves as a cue to caregivers when help
is needed and what kind of help. Normative research in child development suggests that parents who often discuss the causes and consequences of emotion and encourage emotional expression have children
who express higher levels of emotional understanding (Denham and
Grout 1992; Denham et al. 1994). We know that as children BPD patients
did not have this experience. Instead, the parents of the BPD child rarely
discuss emotions, often discourage or punish emotional expression,
and repeatedly misidentify emotional cues and acts toward the child
based on this misunderstanding. Mild misattunement with the child's
intentions attenuates and retards cognitive-emotional integration, but
more extreme misattunment contributes to dissociation and poor cognitive-emotional integration.

The ability to modulate behavior corresponds directly to the child's
level of emotional understanding but also requires consistent parental
assistance. The BPD child, who is hypothesized to have an action-
oriented temperament and is prone toward novelty and excitement
seeking, may need increased parental assistance with regulation. Without an effective goal-corrected partnership, which employs language to
modulate emotion and behavior, both emotion and behavior will become increasingly dysregulated. The child does not learn to replace af-
fect-behavior patterns with symbolic language and executive function

control. Thus, for the BPD patient, both of these developmental lines have gone awry.

Both emotional and behavioral dysregulation are most prominent under threat of neglect, abandonment, or attack. These emotional conditions trigger a collapse and disorganization of the patient's attentional and behavioral strategies for maintaining attachment. When more stably involved in a relationship (i.e., highly preoccupied or maintaining a dismissing/detached form of closeness), the BPD patient's emotions and behaviors are more regulated, and she or he is able to work and maintain routine relationships. These developmental processes are intertwined and expressed within the attachment system. However, over the course of development, both emotional and behavioral dysfunction further maintain and perpetuate the disorder.

INTENSE AND UNSTABLE INTERPERSONAL RELATIONSHIPS

The insecure and disorganized models of attachment and the attendant problems with emotional and behavioral regulation are expressed through intense and unstable adult relationships. BPD patients switch from one mode or self state to another across varying social contexts and exhibit varying degrees of emotional and behavioral dysregulation, depending on their affective experience of interpersonal encounters with significant others.

Examples of how these modes might appear in the therapeutic situation are presented in a schema-focused approach to understanding BPD by Cousineau and Young (1997). These authors propose four schemas: the abandoned child, the detached protector, the punitive parent, and the angry child. The fluctuations among these schemas can be understood as expressions of a disorganized, loosely integrated attachment system. The abandoned or "thrown away" child mode triggers intense affects and frantic behaviors to restore the attachment and bring about equilibrium. In the detached protector mode, a schema of unjust treatment and victimization activates righteous anger, and the patient becomes an "avenging angel" who will right wrongs. This schema is characterized by naïve and overvalued ideas about injustice, right or wrong, and honor and pride. In this mode, the patient attempts to get his or her needs met and to maintain equilibrium through championing the rights of others, often through heroic and unconventional strategies. This may take the form of grievances, lawsuits, or putting one's life on the line. Both the punitive parent and the angry child modes are strategies for maintaining the needed relationship triggered by feelings of maltreatment and usually experienced by others as bullying, controlling, coercive, devious, and manipulative. Another schema that is frequently seen in BPD patients, although not included in the Cousineau and Young's descriptions, is the caretaker mode. BPD patients often function best, albeit at great personal cost, in caretaker roles. In this capacity they maintain attachment through devoted physical and/or psychological care of another.

What is critical to an understanding of patients with BPD is that they are dimly, if at all, conscious of the dramatic shifts in states of mind regarding relationships that are so obvious but puzzling to others. They are, in a sense, surprised by their suddenly shifting emotions and states. Of importance clinically is an understanding of what may trigger these different states of mind and why these patients, unlike others, often cannot remember their behaviors. We propose that their behaviors are activated by fear in response to an experience of maltreatment that triggers the original but now generalized traumatic sensorimotor memories. Each state of mind represents a form of mood state-dependent memory and cannot be retrieved when the person's mood changes. Each mode is activated as a form of stress response to regulate affect and restore safety.

This idea is based on theories of emotion and the role it plays in the encoding, storage, and retrieval of memories. Emotion can be understood as a unit or node in an associative network of concepts (Bower 1981; Clark and Isen 1982). When aroused, an emotion unit becomes associated to events that have been encoded in working memory. Retrieval of memories occurs by supplying one or more activating cues. Retrieval is dependent on state and on context cue, so appropriate retrieval cues are needed for recovery of memories. Evidence suggests that one's emotional state during an event can act as an internal context that becomes part of the complex associated in memory with that event (Bower and Sivers 1998). Emotion is both information and an activator of networks of information.

An example of how BPD patients respond when they feel mistreated illustrates this process. When mistreated, the patient feels helpless, demoralized, and victimized. These feelings activate the patient's generalized early experiences of mistreatment and how she or he learned to respond. The anger and outrage that ensue can trigger a mode of relating characterized by bullying and intimidation. The patient then peremptorily tries to get what she or he needs by coercion. Once the patient is successful and feels secure, this mode of relating disappears and cannot be recalled. Thus, when confronted with her or his behavior, the patient does not accept responsibility for the behavior or explains it as a necessary response to the situation.

Identity Confusion

One's own consciousness or "selfhood" plays a role in organizing and consolidating memories. Memories that can be consciously retrieved are recorded as things that were personally witnessed (Claparède 1911/1995). We highlight here the importance of "witnessing" and "mirroring" in the course of development. A central role of the parent is to witness and voice the child's experience. This serves to develop the sense of a "me" in action across social contexts, bind autobiographical memory, and form identity. The BPD patient had neither an accurate witness nor a "mirror," and this both contributed to and helped to maintain dissociation and prevent consolidation of attachment modes. As a result, memories did not become associated to a continuous "self" at the time of encoding. Because the person has no continuous sense of self, the multiple modes cannot be linked to form a coherent autobiographical memory. The development of a cognitive self and the emergence of autobiographical memory are directly linked to the ability to answer the question "What happened to me?" This cognitive self does not develop until one has a "me" around which to organize it (Howe and Courage 1997), which helps to explain the identity confusion that is another key feature of the disorder.

Intimacy Impediment

The cumulative effect of these multiple developmental problems in the BPD patient is problems with sustained intimacy. BPD, like all personality disorders, is expressed primarily through dysfunctional social relationships and can be understood as a social learning disability. Even though patients with milder forms of the disorder are able to integrate their multiple attachment modes into a more organized preoccupied or dismissing mode, this mode is still an insecure and brittle form of attachment, lacks the flexibility of a secure attachment, and remains vulnerable to disorganization. Thus, true intimacy (i.e., a mutually reciprocal, empathically based relationship) is impeded. Although patients with the most impairment have multiple areas of dysfunction, the most deleterious aspect of the disorder remains the inability to get along and sustain relationships with others. As we will elaborate in subsequent chapters, this feature determines much of the course.

With this explanation of the etiological model, we now turn to its application to the case histories and an explication of how it informs variations in course, outcome, and treatment. We realize that the accuracy and usefulness of the model will have to be tested through future research and clinical application. However, we hope it provides the clinician and researcher with a useful conceptualization with which to articulate etiological hypotheses and to approach treatment and further study.

REFERENCES

Ad-Dab'Bagh Y, Greenfield B: Multiple complex developmental disorder: the "multiple and complex" evolution of the "childhood borderline syndrome" construct. J Am Acad Child Adolesc Psychiatry 40:954–964, 2001

Ainsworth MDS, Wittig MA: Attachment and the exploratory behavior of one-year-olds in a Strange Situation, in Determinants of Infant Behavior, Vol 4. Edited by Foss BM. London, Methuen, 1969, pp pp 111–136

Ainsworth MDS, Blehar MC, Waters E, et al: Patterns of Attachment. Hillsdale, NJ, Erlbaum, 1978

American Psychiatric Association: Diagnostic and Statistical Manual of Mental Disorders, 4th Edition. Washington, DC, American Psychiatric Association, 1994

Andrulonis P, Glueck B, Stroebel C, et al: Organic brain dysfunction and the borderline syndrome. Psychiatr Clin North Am 4:47–66, 1980

Anisman H, Saharia MD, Meaney MJ, et al: Do early life events permanently alter behavioral and hormonal responses to stressors? Int J Dev Neurosci 16: 149–164, 1998

Åsberg M, Träskman L, Thorén P: 5-HIAA in the cerebrospinal fluid: a biochemical suicide predictor? Arch Gen Psychiatry 33:1193–1197, 1976

Baron M, Gruen R, Asnis L, et al: Familial transmission of schizotypal and borderline personality disorders. Am J Psychiatry 142:927–934, 1985

Beeghly M, Cicchetti D: Child maltreatment, attachment, and the self system: emergence of an internal state lexicon in toddlers at high social risk. Dev Psychopathol 6:5–30, 1994

Benoit D, Parker K: Stability and transmission of attachment across three generations. Child Dev 65:1444–1456, 1994

Berg M: Borderline psychopathology as displayed on psychology tests. J Pers Assess 47:120–132, 1983

Bower GH: Mood and memory. Am Psychol 36:129–148, 1981

Bower GH, Sivers H: Cognitive impact of traumatic events. Dev Psychopathol 10:625–653, 1998

Bowlby J: Attachment and Loss, Vol 1: Attachment (1969). New York, Basic Books, 1982

Bowlby J: Attachment and Loss, Vol 2: Separation. New York, Basic Books, 1973

Bowlby J: Attachment and Loss, Vol 3: Loss: Sadness and Depression. London, Hogarth Press/Institute of Psychoanalysis, 1980

Bremner JD, Brett E: Trauma-related dissociative states and long-term psychopathology in posttraumatic stress disorder. J Trauma Stress 10:37–49, 1997

Bremner JD, Krystal JH, Southwick SM, et al: Functioning neuroanatomical correlates of the effects of stress on memory. J Trauma Stress 8:527–553, 1995

Brodsky BS, Oquendo M, Ellis SP, et al: The relationship of childhood abuse to impulsivity and suicidal behavior in adults with major depression. Am J Psychiatry 158:1871–1877, 2001

Cahill L, Haier RJ, Fallon J, et al: Amygdala activity at encoding correlated with long-term free recall of emotional information. Proc Natl Acad Sci 93:8016–8021, 1996

Carlson EA: A prospective longitudinal study of disorganized/disoriented attachment. Child Dev 69:1107–1128, 1998

Carlson V, Cicchetti D, Barnett D, et al: Disorganized/disoriented attachment relationships in maltreated infants. Dev Psychol 25:525–531, 1989

Carpenter C, Gold J, Fenton W: Neuropsychological test results in BPD patients, in 1993 New Research Program and Abstracts, American Psychiatric Association, 146th Annual Meeting, San Francisco, CA, May 12–17, 1993. Washington, DC, American Psychiatric Association, 1993, p 139

Carr A, Goldstein E, Hunt H, et al: Psychological tests and borderline patients. J Pers Assess 43:582–590, 1979

Cassidy J: Theoretical and methodological considerations in the study of attachment and the self in young children, in Attachment in the Preschool Years: Theory, Research and Intervention. Edited by Greenberg MT, Cicchetti D, Cummings EM. Chicago, IL, University of Chicago Press, 1990, pp 87–120

Cheetham SC, Crompton MR, Katona CLE, et al: Brain 5-HT$_2$ receptor binding sites in depressed suicide victims. Brain Res 443:272–280, 1988

Chopra H, Beatson J: Psychotic symptoms in borderline personality disorder. Am J Psychiatry 143:1605–1607, 1986

Cicchetti D, Rogosch FA: Diverse patterns of neuroendocrine activity in maltreated children. Dev Psychopathol 13:677–693, 2001

Cicchetti D, Schneider-Rosen K: Theoretical and empirical consideration in the investigation of the relationship between affect and cognition in atypical populations of infants: contributions to the formulation of an integrative theory of development, in Emotions, Cognition, and Behavior. Edited by Izard C, Kagan J, Zajonc R. New York, Cambridge University Press, 1984, pp 366–406

Cicchetti D, Schneider-Rosen K: An organizational approach to childhood depression, in Depression in Young People: Clinical and Developmental Perspectives. Edited by Rutter M, Izard C, Read P. New York, Guilford, 1986, pp 71–134

Cicchetti D, Tucker D: Development and self-regulatory structures of the mind. Dev Psychopathol 6:533–549, 1994

Cicchetti D, Ackerman BP, Izard C: Emotions and emotion regulation in developmental psychopathology. Dev Psychopathol 7:1–10, 1995

Claparède E: Recognition amoiite. Archive de Psychologie 11:79–90, 1911 [Reprinted, in translation, as "Recognition and Selfhood" in Consciousness and Cognition 4:371–378, 1995]

Clark MS, Isen AM: Towards understanding the relationship between feeling states and social behavior, in Cognitive Social Psychology. Edited by Hastorf A, Isen AM. New York, Elsevier, 1982, pp 73–108

Cloninger CR: A systematic method for clinical description and classification of personality variants. Arch Gen Psychiatry 44:579–588, 1987

Cloninger CR: Temperament and personality. Curr Opin Neurobiol 4:266–273, 1994

Cloninger CR: The psychobiological regulation of social cooperation. Nat Med 1:623–625, 1995

Cloninger C: The genetics and psychobiology of the seven-factor model of personality. Biology of Personality Disorders 17(3):63–92, 1998

Coccaro EF: Central serotonin and impulsive aggression. Br J Psychiatry 155:52–62, 1989

Coccaro EF, Siever LJ, Klar HM, et al: Serotonergic studies in patients with affective and personality disorders: correlates with suicidal and impulsive aggressive behavior. Arch Gen Psychiatry 46:587–599, 1989

Coccaro EF, Bergeman CS, McClearn GE: Heritability of irritable impulsiveness: a study of twins reared together and apart. Psychiatry Res 48:229–242, 1993

Coid J, Petruckevitch A, Feder G, et al: Relation between childhood sexual and physical abuse and risk of revictimisation in women: a cross-sectional survey. Lancet 358:450–454, 2001

Coster W, Gersten MS, Beeghly M, et al: Communicative functioning in maltreated toddlers. Dev Psychol 25:1020–1029, 1989

Cousineau P, Young JE: Treatment of borderline personality disorder with schema-focused approach. Sante Ment Que 22:87–105, 1997

Cowan PA, Cowan CP, Schulz MS: Thinking about risk and resilience in families, in Stress, Coping, and Resiliency in Children and Families. Edited by Hetherington EM, Bleechman EA. Mahwah, NJ, Erlbaum, 1996, pp 1–38

Cowdry RW, Pickar D, Davies R: Symptoms of EEG findings in the borderline syndrome. Int J Psychiatry Med 15:201–211, 1985

Crittenden PM: Internal representational models of attachment relationships. Infant Mental Health Journal 11:259–277, 1990

Dahl AA: Heredity in personality disorders: an overview. Clin Genet 46:138–143, 1994

Damasio A: The Feeling of What Happens. New York, Harcourt Brace, 1999

Debellis MD: Developmental traumatology: the psychobiological development of maltreated children and its implications for research, treatment, and policy. Dev Psychopathol 13:539–564, 2001

Debellis M, Chrousos G, Dorn L, et al: Hypothalamic-pituitary-adrenal axis dysregulation in sexually abused girls. J Clin Endocrinol Metab 7:249–255, 1994

De La Fuente JM, Tugendhaft P, Mavroudakis N: Electroencephalography abnormalities in borderline personality disorder. Psychiatry Res 77:131–138, 1998

Denham SA, Grout L: Mother's emotional expressiveness and coping: relations with preschoolers' social-emotional competence. Genetic, Social and General Psychology Monographs 118(1):73–101, 1992

Denham SA, Zoller D, Couchoud EA: Socialization of preschoolers emotional understanding. Dev Psychol 30:928–936, 1994

Derryberry D, Rothbart MK: Reactive and effortful processes in the organization of temperament. Dev Psychopathol 9:633–652, 1997

Digman JM: Personality structure: emergence of the five-factor model. Annu Rev Psychol 50:116–123, 1990

Driessen M, Herrmann J, Stahl K, et al: Magnetic resonance imaging volumes of the hippocampus amygdala in women with borderline personality disorder and early traumatization. Arch Gen Psychiatry 57:1115–1122, 2000

Dube SR, Anda RF, Felitti VJ, et al: Childhood abuse, household dysfunction, and the risk of attempted suicide throughout the life span. JAMA 286:3089–3096, 2001

Exner JE: Some Rorschach data comparing schizophrenics with borderline and schizotypal personality disorders. J Pers Assess 50:455–471, 1986

Flavell JH: Metacognition and cognitive monitoring: a new area of cognitive-developmental inquiry. Am Psychol 34:906–911, 1979

Flavell JH, Flavell ER, Green FL: Development of the appearance-reality distinction. Cognitive Psychology 15:95–120, 1983

Foa EB, Riggs DS, Gershuny BS: Arousal, numbing, and intrusion: symptom structure of PTSD following assault. Am J Psychiatry 152:116–120, 1995

Fonagy P, Leigh T, Steele M, et al: The relationship of attachment status, psychiatric classification, and response to psychotherapy. J Consult Clin Psychol 64:22–31, 1996

Fonagy P, Target M, Gergely G: Attachment and borderline personality disorder: a theory and some evidence. Psychiatr Clin North Am 23:103–122, 2000

Forguson L, Gopnik A: The ontogeny of common sense, in Developing Theories of Mind. Edited by Astington JW, Harris PL, Olson DR. New York, Cambridge University Press, 1988, pp 226–243

Fossati A, Madeddu F, Maffei C: Borderline personality disorder and childhood sexual abuse: a meta-analytic study. J Personal Disord 13:268–280, 1999

Fyer MF, Frances AJ, Sullivan T, et al: Comorbidity of borderline personality disorder. Arch Gen Psychiatry 45:348–352, 1988

Gardner D, Lucas PB, Cowdry RW: Soft sign neurological abnormalities in borderline personality disorder and normal control subjects. J Nerv Ment Dis 175:77–180, 1987

George A, Soloff P: Schizotypal symptoms of inpatients with borderline personality disorder. Am J Psychiatry 143:212–215, 1986

George C, Kaplan N, Main M: Adult Attachment Interview Protocol. Unpublished manuscript, University of California, Berkeley, 1984

George C, Kaplan N, Main M: Adult Attachment Interview Protocol, 2nd Edition. Unpublished manuscript, University of California, Berkeley, 1985

George C, Kaplan N, Main M: Adult Attachment Interview Protocol, 3rd Edition. Unpublished manuscript, University of California, Berkeley, 1996

Gibb BE, Wheeler R, Alloy LB, et al: Emotional, physical, and sexual maltreatment in childhood versus adolescence and personality dysfunction in young adulthood. J Personal Disord 15:505–511, 2001

Gladstone G, Parker G, Wilhelm K, et al: Characteristics of depressed patients who report childhood sexual abuse. Am J Psychiatry 156:431–437, 1999

Glaser D: Child abuse and neglect and the brain: a review. J Child Psychol Psychiatry 41:97–116, 2000

Goldsmith H, Alansky JA: Maternal and infant temperamental predictors of attachment: a meta-analytic review. J Consult Clin Psychol 55:805–816, 1987

Goldsmith HH, Buss AH, Plomin R: What is temperament? Four approaches. Child Dev 58:505–529, 1987

Gunderson J: Borderline Personality Disorder. Washington, DC, American Psychiatric Press, 1984

Gunderson J, Sabo AN: The phenomenological and conceptual interface between borderline personality disorder and PTSD. Am J Psychiatry 150:19–27, 1993

Gunderson J, Zanarini M: Pathogenesis of borderline personality disorder, in American Psychiatric Press Review of Psychiatry, Vol 8. Edited by Tasman A, Hales R, Frances A. Washington, DC, American Psychiatric Press, 1989, pp 25–48

Gunderson J, Kerr J, Englund D: The families of borderlines: a comparative study. Arch Gen Psychiatry 37:27–33, 1980

Guzder J, Paris J, Zelkowitz P, et al: Psychological risk factors for borderline pathology in school-age children. J Am Acad Child Adolesc Psychiatry 38:206–212, 1999

Herman J, Perry C, van der Kolk B: Childhood trauma in borderline personality disorder. Am J Psychiatry 146:490–495, 1989

Hesse E: The Adult Attachment Interview: historical and current perspectives, in Handbook of Attachment. Edited by Cassidy J, Shaver PR, Main M. New York, Guilford, 1999, pp 395–433

Hesse E, Main M: Disorganized infant, child, and adult attachment: collapse in behavioral and attentional strategies. J Am Psychoanal Assoc 48:1097–1127, 2000

Howe MS, Courage ML: The emergence and early development of autobiographical memory. Psychol Rev 104:499–523, 1997

Izard CE: The structure and functions of emotions: implications for cognition, motivation, and personality, in The G Stanley Hall Lecture Series, Vol 9. Edited by Cohen IS. Washington, DC, American Psychological Association, 1989, pp 39–73

Johnson DM, Shea MT, Yen S, et al: Gender differences in borderline personality disorder: findings from the Collaborative Longitudinal Personality Disorders Study (submitted for publication)

Johnson JG, Cohen P, Brown J, et al: Childhood maltreatment increases risk for personality disorders during early adulthood. Arch Gen Psychiatry 56:600–606, 1999

Judd P, Ruff R: Neuropsychological dysfunction in borderline personality disorder. J Personal Disord 7:275–284, 1993

Kaplan ML, Asnis GM, Lipschitz DS, et al: Suicidal behavior and abuse in psychiatric outpatients. Compr Psychiatry 36:229–235, 1995

Kendler KS, Bulik CM, Silberg J, et al: Childhood sexual abuse and adult psychiatric and substance use disorders in women. Arch Gen Psychiatry 57: 953–959, 2000

Kernberg O: Borderline personality organization. J Am Psychoanal Assoc 15: 641–685, 1967

Kernberg O: Borderline Conditions and Pathological Narcissism. New York, Jason Aronson, 1975

Kimble CR, Oepen G, Weinberg E, et al: Neurological vulnerability and trauma in borderline personality disorder, in Role of Sexual Abuse in the Etiology of Borderline Personality Disorder. Edited by Zanarini MC. Washington, DC, American Psychiatric Press, 1997, pp 165–180

Korpi ER, Klineman JE, Goodman SI, et al: Serotonin and 5-hydroxyindoleacetic acid concentrations in brains of suicide victims: comparison in chronic schizophrenic patients with suicide as cause of death. Arch Gen Psychiatry 43:594–600, 1986

Krystal JH, Southwick SM, Charney DS: Posttraumatic stress disorder: psychobiological mechanisms of traumatic remembrance, in Memory Distortion: How Minds, Brains, and Societies Reconstruct the Past. Edited by Schacter D. Cambridge, MA, Harvard University Press, 1995, pp 150–172

Kutcher SP, Blackwood DHK, St. Clair D, et al: Auditory P300 in borderline personality disorder and schizophrenia. Arch Gen Psychiatry 44:645–650, 1987

Lai ZC: A proposed neural circuitry underlying the processing of emotional cues derived from a syndrome of social skill impairment: a functional evolutionary architectonic perspective. Special Area Paper. Minneapolis, Clinical Psychology Program, University of Minnesota, 1990

Lane RD, Schwartz GD: Levels of emotional awareness: a cognitive-developmental theory and its application to psychopathology. Am J Psychiatry 144: 133–143, 1987

Lincoln AJ, Bloom D, Katz M, et al: Neuropsychological and neurophysiological indices of auditory processing impairment in children with multiple complex developmental disorder. J Am Acad Child Adolesc Psychiatry 35:100–112, 1998

Linehan MM: Cognitive-Behavioral Treatment of Borderline Personality Disorder. New York, Guilford, 1993

Linehan MM: Understanding Borderline Personality Disorder. New York, Guilford, 1995

Links PS, Steiner M, Huxley G: The occurrence of borderline personality disorder in the families of borderline patients. J Personal Disord 2:14–20, 1988

Links PS, Boggild A, Sarin N: Modeling the relationship between affective lability, impulsivity, and suicidal behavior in patients with borderline personality disorder. Journal of Psychiatric Practice 6:247–255, 2000

Linnoila M, Virkkunen M, Scheinin M, et al: Low cerebrospinal fluid 5-hydroxyindoleacetic acid concentration differentiates impulsive from nonimpulsive violent behavior. Life Sci 33:2609–2614, 1983

Linotti G: Disorganization of attachment as a model for understanding dissociative psychopathology, in Attachment Disorganization. Edited by Solomon J, George C. London, Guilford, 1999, pp 291–317

Livesley WJ, Jang KL, Jackson DN, et al: Genetic and environmental contributions to dimensions of personality disorder. Am J Psychiatry 150:1826–1831, 1993

López-Ibor JJ, Lana F, Saiz Ruiz J: Impulsive suicidal behavior and serotonin. Actas Luso Esp Neurol Psiquiatr Cienc Afines 18:316–325, 1990

Luria A: The Working Brain. New York, Basic Books, 1973

Luria A: Higher Cortical Functions in Man, 2nd Edition. Translated by Haigh B. New York, Basic Books, 1980

Lyons-Ruth K, Block D: The disturbed caregiving system: relations among childhood trauma, maternal caregiving and infant affect and attachment. Infant Mental Health Journal 17:257–275, 1996

Lyoo IK, Han MH, Cho DY: A brain MRI study in subjects with borderline personality disorder. J Affect Disord 50:235–243, 1998

Macfie J, Cicchetti D, Toth SL: The development of dissociation in maltreated preschool-aged children. Dev Psychopathol 13:233–254, 2001

MacMillan HL, Fleming JE, Streiner DL, et al: Childhood abuse and lifetime psychopathology in a community sample. Am J Psychiatry 158:1878–1883, 2001

Main M: Metacognitive knowledge, metacognitive monitoring, and singular (coherent) vs multiple (incoherent) models of attachment: findings and directions for future research, in Attachment Across the Life Cycle. Edited by Marris P, Stevenson-Hinde J, Parkes C. New York, Routledge, 1991, pp 127–159

Main M: The organized catergories of infant, child, and adult attachment: flexible vs inflexible attention under attachment-related stress. J Am Psychoanal Assoc 48:1055–1096, 2000

Main M, Hesse E: Parents' unresolved traumatic experiences are related to infant disorganized attachment status: is frightened and/or frightening parental behavior the linking mechanism? in Attachment in the Preschool Years: Theory, Research and Intervention. Edited by Greenberg M, Cicchetti D, Cummings EM. Chicago, IL. University of Chicago Press, 1990, pp 161–184

Main M, Solomon J: Procedures for identifying infants as disorganized/disoriented during the Ainsworth Strange Situation, in Attachment in the Preschool Years: Theory, Research and Intervention. Edited by Greenberg M, Cicchetti D, Cummings EM. Chicago, IL. University of Chicago Press, 1990, pp 121–160

Main M, Kaplan N, Cassidy J: Security in infancy, childhood, and adulthood: a move to the level of representation, in Growing Points of Attachment: Theory and Research (Monogr Soc Res Child Dev, No 209, Vol 50 [1–2]). Edited by Bretherton I, Waters E. Chicago, IL, University of Chicago Press, 1985, pp 66–104

Malatesta-Magai C: Emotional socialization: its role in personality and developmental psychopathology, in Internalizing and Externalizing Expressions of Dysfunction (Rochester Symposium on Developmental Psychology). Edited by Cicchetti D, Toth SL. Hillsdale, NJ, Erlbaum, 1991, pp 203–224

Mann JJ, Stanley M, McBride PA, et al: Increased serotonin₂ and β-adrenergic receptor binding in the frontal cortices of suicide victims. Arch Gen Psychiatry 43:954–959, 1986

Marshall RD, Olfson M, Hellman F, et al: Comorbidity, impairment, and suicidality in subthreshold PTSD. Am J Psychiatry 158:1467–1473, 2001

Masterson J, Rinsley D: The borderline syndrome: the role of the mother in the genesis and psychic structure of the borderline personality. Int J Psychoanal 56:163–177, 1975

McClelland JL, McNaughton BL, O'Reilly RC: Why there are complementary learning systems in the hippocampus and neocortex: insights from the successes and failures of connectionist models of learning and memory. Psychol Rev 102:419–457, 1995

McCrae RR, Costa PT Jr: Personality in Adulthood. New York, Guilford. 1990

McCrae RR, John OP: An introduction to the five-factor model and its applications. J Pers 54:430–446, 1992

McGlashan TH, Grilo CM, Skodol AE: The Collaborative Longitudinal Personality Disorders Study: baseline Axis I/II and II/II diagnostic co-occurrence. Acta Psychiatr Scand 102:256–264, 2000

Meaney M J, Diorio J, Francis D, et al: Early environmental regulation of forebrain glucocorticoid receptor gene expression: implications for adrenocortical responses to stress. Dev Neurosci 18:49–72, 1996

Meltzer HY, Perline R, Tricou BJ, et al: Effect of 5-hydroxytryptophan on serum cortisol levels in major affective disorders, II: relation to suicide, psychosis, and depressive symptoms. Arch Gen Psychiatry 46:587–599, 1984

Meyer SE, Chrousos GP, Gold PW: Major depression and the stress system: a life span perspective. Dev Psychopathol 13:565–580, 2001

Newmark C, Sines L: Characteristics of hospitalized patients who produced the "floating" MMPI profiles. J Clin Psychol 28:74–76, 1972

Nigg JT, Silk KR, Westen D, et al: Object representations in early memories of sexually abused borderline patients. Am J Psychiatry 148:864–869, 1991

O'Connell M, Cooper S, Perry J, et al: The relationship between thought disorder and psychotic symptoms in borderline personality disorder. J Nerv Ment Dis 177:273–278, 1989

Ogata SN, Silk KR, Goodrich S, et al: Childhood sexual and physical abuse in adult patients with borderline personality disorder. Am J Psychiatry 147:1008–1013, 1990

Ogawa JR, Sroufe LA, Weinfield NS, et al: Development and the fragmented self: longitudinal study of dissociative symptomatology in a nonclinical sample. Dev Psychopathol 9:855–879, 1997

O'Leary K, Brouwers P, Gardner D, et al: Neuropsychological testing of patients with borderline personality disorder. Am J Psychiatry 148:106–111, 1991

Palombo J: Psychodynamic and relational problems of children with nonverbal learning disabilities, in Handbook of Infant, Child and Adolescent Psychotherapy: Guide to Diagnosis and Treatment. Edited by Mark B, Incorvaia J. New York, Jason Aronson, 1995, pp 147–178

Paris J: Predispositions, personality traits, and posttraumatic stress disorder. Harv Rev Psychiatry 8(4):175–183, 2000

Paris J, Zweig-Frank H, Guzder H: The role of psychological risk factors in recovery from borderline personality disorder. Compr Psychiatry 34:410–413, 1993

Paris J, Zelkowitz J, Guzder J, et al: Neuropsychological factors associated with borderline pathology in children. J Am Acad Child Adolesc Psychiatry 38: 770–774, 1999

Parker G, Hadzi-Pavlovic D, Wilhelm K: Modeling and measuring the personality disorders. Journal of Personality Disorders 14:189–198, 2000

Patrick J: Characteristics of DSM-III borderline MMPI profiles. J Clin Psychol 40: 655–658, 1984

Patrick M, Hobson RP, Castle D, et al: Personality disorder and the mental representation of early social experience. Dev Psychopathol 6:375–388, 1994

Pine F: On the development of the "borderline-child-to-be." Am J Orthopsychiatry 56:450–457, 1986

Pope HG Jr, Jonas JM, Hudson JI, et al: An empirical study of psychosis in borderline personality disorder. Am J Psychiatry 142:1285–1290, 1985

Putnam FW: Dissociative disorders in children: behavioral profiles and problems. Child Abuse Negl 17:39–45, 1993

Quitkin F, Rifkin A, Klein D: Neurological soft signs in schizophrenia and character disorders. Arch Gen Psychiatry 33:845–853, 1976

Rieber R, Carton AS (eds): The Collected Works of L. S. Vygotsky, Vol 1: Problems of General Psychology. New York, Plenum, 1987, pp 326

Rinne T, Westerberg HG, den Boer JA, et al: Serotonergic blunting to meta-chlorophenylpiperazine (m-CPP) highly correlates with sustained childhood abuse in impulsive and auto-aggressive female born patients. Biol Psychiatry 47:548–556, 2000

Romans SE, Martin JL, Morris E, et al: Psychological defense styles in women who report childhood sexual abuse: a controlled community study. Am J Psychiatry 156:1080–1085, 1999

Rothbart MK, Bates JE: Temperament, in Handbook of Child Psychology, 5th Edition, Vol 3: Social, Emotional and Personality Development. Edited by Damon W, Eisenberg N. New York, Wiley, 1998

Sameroff AJ, Chandler MJ: Reproductive risk and the continuum of caretaking casualty, in Review of Child Development Research, Vol 4. Edited by In Horowitz FD. Chicago, IL, University of Chicago Press, 1975, pp 187–244

Sameroff AJ, Fiese BH: Transactional regulation and early intervention, in Handbook of Early Childhood Intervention. Edited by Meisels SJ, Shonkoff JP. New York, Cambridge University Press, 1990, pp 119–149

Sameroff AJ, Fiese BH: Models of development and developmental risk, in Handbook of Infant Mental Health, 2nd Edition. Edited by Zeanah CH. New York, Guilford, 2000, pp 3–19

Sanislow CA, Grilo CM, McGlashan TH: Factor analysis of the DSM-III-R borderline personality criteria in psychiatric inpatients. Am J Psychiatry 157: 1629–1633, 2000

Sanislow CA, Grilo CM, Morey LC, et al: Confirmatory factor analysis of DSM-IV criteria for borderline personality disorder: findings from the Collaborative Longitudinal Personality Disorders Study. Am J Psychiatry 159:284–290, 2002

Shapiro E, Zinner J, Shapiro R: The influence of family experience on borderline personality development. Int Rev Psychoanal 2:399–411, 1975

Siever LS, Davis KL: A psychobiologic perspective on the personality disorders. Am J Psychiatry 148:1647–1658, 1991

Siever LJ, Trestman RL: The serotonin system and aggressive personality disorder. Internationl Journal of Clinical Psychopharmacology 8(2):33–39, 1993

Silk K, Lohr N, Westen D, et al: Psychosis in borderline patients with depression. Journal of Personality Disorders 3:92–100, 1989

Singer MI, Petchers MK, Hussey D: The relationship between sexual abuse and substance abuse among psychiatrically hospitalized adolescents. Child Abuse Negl 13:319–325, 1989

Singer MT: The borderline diagnosis and psychological tests: review and research, in Borderline Personality Disorders: The Concept, the Syndrome. Edited by Hartocollis P. New York, International Universities Press, 1977, pp 193–212

Singer MT, Larson DG: Borderline personality and the Rorschach test. Arch Gen Psychiatry 38:693–698, 1981

Sjöberg RL, Lindbland F: Limited disclosure of sexual abuse in children whose experiences were documented by videotape. Am J Psychiatry 159:312–314, 2002

Snyder S, Pitts W: Electroencephalography of DSM-III borderline personality disorder. Acta Psychiatr Scand 69:129–134, 1984

Soloff PH, Millward JW: Developmental histories of borderline patients. Compr Psychiatry 24:574–588, 1983

Soloff PH, Lynch KG, Kelly TM, et al: Characteristics of suicide attempts of patients with major depressive episode and borderline personality disorder: a comparative study. Am J Psychiatry 157:601–608, 2000

Southwick SM, Yehuda R, Giller Jr EL: Personality disorders in treatment-seeking combat veterans with posttraumatic stress disorder. Am J Psychiatry 150: 1020–1023, 1993

Spangler G, Grossmann KE: Biobehavioral organization in securely and insecurely attached infants. Child Dev 64:1439–1450, 1993

Sroufe LA: Socioemotional development, in Handbook of Infant Development. Edited by Osofsky J. New York, Wiley, 1979, pp 462–516

Sroufe LA, Fleeson J: The coherence of family relationships, in Relationships Within Families: Mutual Influences. Edited by Hinde R, Stevenson-Hinde J. Oxford, UK, Clarendon, 1988, pp 27–47

Sroufe LA, Rutter M: The domain of developmental psychopathology. Child Dev 55:17–29, 1984

Stanley B, Molcho A, Stanley M, et al: Association of aggressive behavior with altered serotonergic function in patients who are not suicidal. Am J Psychiatry 157:609–614, 2000

Stein M, Koverola C, Hanna C, et al: Hippocampal volume in women victimized by childhood sexual abuse. Psychol Med 27:951–959, 1997

Stern DN: The Interpersonal World of the Infant: A View From Psychoanalysis and Developmental Psychology. New York, Basic Books, 1985

Sternbach S, Judd P, Sabo A, et al: Cognitive and perceptual distortions in borderline personality disorder and schizotypal personality disorder in a vignette sample. Compr Psychiatry 33:186–189, 1992

Strick FL, Wilcox SA: A comparison of dissociative experiences in adult female outpatients with and without histories of early incestuous abuse. Dissociation 4:193–199, 1991

Sugarman A: The borderline personality organization as manifested on psychological tests, in Borderline Phenomena and the Rorschach Test. Edited by Kwawer J, Lerner H, Lerner D, et al. New York, International Universities Press, 1980, pp 39–57

Swirsky-Sacchetti T, Gorton G, Samuel S, et al: Neuropsychological function in borderline personality disorder. J Clin Psychol 49:385–396, 1993

Torgersen S: Genetics in borderline conditions. Acta Psychiatr Scand Suppl 379: 19–25, 1994

Torgersen S: Genetics of patients with borderline personality disorder. Psychiatr Clin North Am 23:1–9, 2000

Torgersen S, Lygren S, Oien PA, et al: A twin study of personality disorders. Compr Psychiatry 41:416–425, 2000

Towbin KE, Dykens EM, Pearson GS, et al: Conceptualizing "borderline syndrome of childhood" and "childhood schizophrenia" as a developmental disorder. J Am Acad Child Adolesc Psychiatry 32:775–782, 1993

van IJzendoorn MH: Adult attachment representations, parental responsiveness, and infant attachment: a meta-analysis on the predictive validity of the Adult Attachment Interview. Psychol Bull 117:387–403, 1995

van IJzendoorn MH, Goldberg S, Kroonenberg PM, et al: The relative effects of maternal and child problems on the quality of attachment: a meta-analysis of attachment in clinical samples. Child Dev 63:840–858, 1992

van IJzendoorn MH, Schuengel C, Bakermans-Kranenburg MJ: Disorganized attachment in early childhood: meta-analysis of precursors, concomitants, and sequelae. Dev Psychopathol 11:225–249, 1999

Van Reekum R, Conway CA, Gansler D, et al: Neurobehavioral study of borderline personality disorder. J Psychiatry Neurosci 18:121–129, 1993

Verkes RJ, Van der Mast RC, Kerkhof AJ, et al: Platelet serotonin, monoamine oxidase activity, and [^{3}H]paroxetine binding related to impulsive suicide attempts and borderline personality disorder. Biol Psychiatry 43:740–746, 1998

Waldinger RJ, Swett C, Frank A, et al: Levels of dissociation and histories of reported abuse among women outpatients. J Nerv Ment Dis 182:625–630, 1994

Waller N, Putnam FW, Carlson EB: Types of dissociation and dissociative types: a taxometric analysis of dissociative experiences. Psychological Methods 1:300–321, 1996

Wechsler D: The Measurement and Appraisal of Adult Intelligence, 4th Edition. Baltimore, MD, Williams & Wilkins, 1958

Weschler D: Wechsler Adult Intelligence Scale—Revised Manual. New York, Psychological Corporation/Harcourt, Brace, Jovanovich, 1981

Widiger TA: Psychological tests and the borderline diagnosis. J Pers Assessment 46:227–238, 1982

Widiger TA, Trull TJ, Clarkin JF, et al: A description of the DSM-III-R and DSM-IV personality disorder with the five-factor model of personality, in Personality Disorders and the Five-Factor Model of Personality. Edited by Costa PT, Widiger TA. Washington, DC, American Psychological Association, 1994, pp 41–56

Wonderlich SA, Crosby RD, Mitchell JE, et al: Sexual trauma and personality: developmental vulnerability and additive effects. Journal of Personality Disorders 15:496–504, 2001

Yen S, Battle CL, Johnson DM, et al: Traumatic exposure and posttraumatic stress disorder in borderline, schizotypal, avoidant and obsessive-compulsive personality disorders: findings from the Collaborative Longitudinal Personality Disorders Study (submitted for publication)

Zanarini MC (ed): Role of Sexual Abuse in the Etiology of Borderline Personality Disorder. Washington, DC, American Psychiatric Press, 1997

Zanarini M, Gunderson JG, Marino MF, et al: DSM-III disorders in the families of borderline outpatients. Journal of Personality Disorders 2:292–302, 1988

Zanarini MC, Gunderson J, Marino M, et al: Childhood experiences of borderline patients. Compr Psychiatry 30:18–25, 1989

Zanarini MC, Gunderson J, Frankenburg F: Cognitive features of borderline personality disorder. Am J Psychiatry 147:57–63, 1990

Zanarini MC, Williams AA, Lewis RE, et al: Reported pathological childhood experiences associated with the development of borderline personality disorder. Am J Psychiatry 154:1101–1106, 1997

Zanarini MC, Ruser TF, Frankenburg FR, et al: Related factors associated with the dissociative experiences of borderline patients. J Nerv Ment Dis 188:26–30, 2000

Zinner J, Shapiro E: Splitting in families of borderline adolescents, in Borderline States in Psychiatry. Edited by Mack J. New York, Grune & Stratton, 1975, pp 103–122

Zlotnick C, Zimmerman M, Wolfsdorf BA, et al: Gender differences in patients with posttraumatic stress disorder in a general psychiatric practice. Am J Psychiatry 158:1923–1925, 2001

Zweig-Frank H, Paris J, Guzder J: Dissociation in female patients with borderline and non-borderline personality disorders. Journal of Personality Disorders 8:203–209, 1994a

Zweig-Frank H, Paris J, Guzder J: Dissociation in male patients with borderline and non-borderline personality disorders. Journal of Personality Disorders 8:210–218, 1994b

II

Variations in Course and Outcome: Case Histories

2

The Chestnut Lodge
Follow-Up Study

Time present and time past
Are both perhaps present in time future,
And time future contained in time past.

T. S. Eliot, "Burnt Norton" (Four Quartets)

CHESTNUT LODGE: TREATMENT
SETTING AND PHILOSOPHY

The patients described in the next four chapters were patients at Chestnut Lodge Hospital between 1950 and 1975. At that time, American psychiatry was primarily psychoanalytically and/or psychodynamically oriented yet undergoing the early phases of a paradigmatic shift to biological psychiatry, with its focus on reliable diagnosis and pharmacotherapy. The diagnostic classification systems existing during this period were DSM-I (American Psychiatric Association 1952) and DSM-II (American Psychiatric Association 1968). Medication treatment consisted primarily of chlorpromazine and similar neuroleptics for psychotic disorders. Pharmacotherapy was in its infancy, with the introduction of tricyclic antidepressants and the mood stabilizer lithium carbonate. These psychodynamic and biological trends were not integrated theoretically. In practice, they coexisted precariously—often competitively. At the time in question, Chestnut Lodge was clearly in the camp of mind, not brain, and the march of molecules into the consulting room was usually viewed by the professional staff as an antitherapeutic invasion and narcissistic assault.

In 1960 Chestnut Lodge had been a psychiatric hospital for 50 years, having been opened in 1910 by Ernest Bullard, M.D., a psychiatrist from the Midwest. He converted what had been a resort hotel in Rockville, MD, into a hospital, largely for the care and treatment of patients with alcoholism and senile dementia. His son, Dexter Bullard Sr., M.D., inherited the hospital and medical directorship in the 1920s. His interest and training in psychoanalysis and in psychosis, coupled with the fortuitous arrival of Frieda Fromm-Reichmann in the 1930s, led to the transformation of the institution into its unique and now timeless place in American psychiatry as a center for the practice and teaching of intensive psychoanalytically oriented psychotherapy of patients with severe mental illness.

At the time these patients were treated, Chestnut Lodge was a family-owned and family-run inpatient psychiatric institution. Dexter Bullard Sr., M.D., was the medical director from 1931 to 1968, at which time his eldest son, Dexter Bullard Jr., M.D., took the helm as medical director and chairman of the family-run board of directors. He, too, was a psychiatrist and psychoanalyst, and he directed the institution until his death in 1995.

The "golden era" of Chestnut Lodge probably spans the period of Freida Fromm-Reichmann's tenure at the institution, from 1935 to 1958, when she served as director of psychotherapy and lived on the grounds of the institution in a cottage built for her by Dexter Bullard Sr., and where she saw analysands, supervisees, and patients, including Joanna Goldenberg of *I Never Promised You a Rose Garden* fame. In her seminal work *Principles of Intensive Psychotherapy,* Fromm-Reichmann (1950/1960) championed a paradigmatic shift of American psychiatry into the application of using psychodynamic psychotherapy for all manner of psychiatric disorders. During the period of her tenure, many notables of mid-Atlantic American psychiatry, such as Harry Stack Sullivan, Otto Will, Robert Cohen, Harold Searles, Alfred Stanton, and Marvin Schwartz, had contact with Chestnut Lodge as trainees, medical staff members, consultants, or visitors.

Rockville, MD, where Chestnut Lodge was located, was, during the period in question, a small middle- and lower-middle-class town that was rapidly becoming a near suburb of Washington, DC. The Lodge was spread across 100 pastoral acres of wooded lawns and open grassy fields. Its name derived from a collection of magnificent American chestnut trees that had disappeared in the chestnut blight earlier in the century. It housed approximately 100 patients in four buildings and seven units, five that were locked and two that were open. Each unit housed 10–15 patients. None of the buildings had been erected as psychiatric units; the grounds and buildings originally served as a resort hotel, mostly for nearby Washingtonians who wished to escape the bustle and heat of that swampy, pre-air-conditioned city. The grounds also held a dining hall and adjoining recreation center; an office building for the medical staff, with a basement library/meeting room; and two residences, Dr. Fromm-Reichmann's cottage and Dr. Bullard's home and office.

Chestnut Lodge was a tertiary care psychiatric hospital, admitting patients who were severely ill and who usually had an established history of treatment failure at other private psychiatric facilities in America, especially on the eastern seaboard. Approximately 60% of the patients had schizophrenia or schizoaffective disorder, 20% had borderline and other personality disorders, and 20% had a mixture of affective disorders and character pathology. Virtually all patients were from upper-middle-class or upper-class families and were self-paying. Insurance coverage was at least a generation in the future. The average length of stay was 2 years.

The treatment for all patients was intensive psychoanalytically oriented psychotherapy, usually 50 minutes in length, four to five times per week. It was conducted in the therapist's office in the medical staff building, unless the patient was too psychotic or out of control to leave her or his unit, in which case the therapist came to the unit for the "hour." If necessary, the patient was seen in restraints, usually sheet pack.

Psychoactive drugs were seldom used. Psychotic patients were usually withdrawn from neuroleptics on admission and placed back on these agents only if their psychosis failed to respond to 1–2 years of psychotherapy alone. Antipsychotic medication, when used, was restricted to psychotic patients. Tricyclic antidepressants and lithium, although emergent in the late 1960s and 1970s, were not used as such. The treatment of patients with BPD at Chestnut Lodge during this time consisted exclusively of intensive psychotherapy plus the standard collection of adjunctive occupational and recreational therapies.

The treatment model at Chestnut Lodge incorporated the so-called T-A split, or therapist-administrator team. Each patient was under the care of two doctors. The therapist provided psychotherapy, and the administrator ran the unit on which the patient lived and was responsible for all day-to-day decisions regarding the patient's care, such as privileges, restrictions, physical health, and medications (if any). In the period of time in question, all therapists and administrators were full-time members of the Chestnut Lodge Medical Staff, all were M.D.s and psychiatrists, and most were psychoanalysts or in psychoanalytic training.

The treatment process at Chestnut Lodge was fairly uniform, if not ritualized. After admission, the patient would undergo an extensive evaluation, including the compiling of their usually voluminous past records; a psychiatric and physical evaluation; a psychological assessment, typically consisting of the Wechsler Adult Intelligence Test, the Rorschach, the Thematic Apperception Test, and a Bender-Gestalt; and an introduction to intensive psychotherapy. After about 2 months, the patient's case would be presented to the entire medical staff by the therapist and the administrator. The history of illness was detailed, a diagnosis decided, and a dynamic formulation offered to guide the now ongoing psychotherapy. A different therapist or unit (and administrator) could be chosen at this point, but such an occurrence was uncommon. As the psychotherapy proceeded, the patient would participate in a variety of "activities." These activities were either localized to her or his unit, as with community meetings, or located in other buildings on the grounds, as with occupational therapy.

The patient's treatment and progress were reviewed in three ways. First, a more experienced member of the medical staff almost always supervised the psychotherapist's work with the patient. Second, the medical staff split up into small subgroups of five or six members and met for 1½ hours twice each week to discuss work with patients in an unstructured format. Finally, the medical staff met as a whole for 2 hours once a week to review the work of a single patient. The primary focus was on the psychotherapy, with the therapist presenting his or her work with the patient in some detail, along with representative examples of treatment sessions. Starting in 1941 this exercise was routinely transcribed, and it is largely from these verbatim transcripts that the case histories presented in this book were reconstructed.

As patients progressed in their stay at Chestnut Lodge, they would occasionally move off grounds into Rockville or the surrounding territory and continue with their Lodge therapist as an outpatient. More often, when this point was reached, they would return closer to home, whether or not they had plans to continue treatment. Patients failing to progress would often remain at Chestnut Lodge for years or be transferred to a private or public inpatient facility closer to their home.

The long-term (15-year) outcome of the majority of patients treated at Chestnut Lodge between 1950 and 1975 has been tracked, documented, and published (McGlashan 1984a, 1984b, 1986). Overall, patients with psychosis did poorly, patients with affective disorders made minimal to moderate progress, and patients with BPD did reasonably well. We hope to illustrate the range of outcomes that characterize the borderline group and to speculate as to the forces determining this heterogeneity.

CHESTNUT LODGE FOLLOW-UP STUDY

Long-Term Course and Outcome of BPD at Chestnut Lodge

The longitudinal study of BPD was part of a larger, comprehensive investigation of all patients treated at Chestnut Lodge, most of whom had schizophrenia, an affective disorder, or the borderline disorder. The follow-up study's design and methodology have been elaborated in detail elsewhere (McGlashan 1984a, 1984b). Briefly, the study was retrospective and incorporated six elements to ensure methodologic rigor:

- Operationally defined diagnostic criteria
- Adequate demographic and predictor characterization of samples
- Multidimensionally measured outcome
- Independence of follow-up data collection from the baseline diagnostic and demographic and predictor data collection
- Reliability testing of all measures
- Bias testing of missing subject subsamples

Included in the follow-up study were 454 patients discharged from the hospital between 1950 and 1975 and a smaller cohort of nondischarged inpatients from a comparable period. Selected were those without organic brain syndrome who were between 16 and 55 years of age on admission and who were treated at Chestnut Lodge for a minimum of 90 days. Two realms of data were of interest—outcome and baseline diagnostic/demographic—the evaluations of which were conducted independently.

Outcome data were collected, following informed consent, an average of 15 years after discharge (range = 2 to 32 years) via interviews with the subjects and/or significant others. The majority of interviews were conducted by telephone and averaged 2 hours in length.

For baseline diagnostic and demographic assessment, the voluminous index hospitalization medical records were transposed onto a 25-page document called the Chart Abstract, which was used to rate each patient on many demographic/predictor and sign and symptom variables. On the basis of these abstracted clinical data, all patients were scored according to current diagnostic systems. The diagnoses of schizophrenia, bipolar affective disorder, and unipolar affective disorder were given to any patient satisfying DSM-III criteria for these disorders. The diagnosis of borderline was given to any patient meeting either the DSM-III criteria for BPD or the Gunderson and Kolb criteria for borderline disorder (Gunderson and Kolb 1978).

Outcome of BPD Compared With Axis I Disorders

A substantial number ($N = 81$) of patients were diagnosed with BPD. The overall findings related to BPD are summarized elsewhere (Mc-Glashan 1992), and parts of that summary are reproduced here. To place BPD outcome within a larger and well-informed perspective, we compared our BPD patients with patients from the follow-up study with schizophrenia and unipolar affective disorder (McGlashan 1986).

Figure 2–1 schematically summarizes the frequency distribution of the global clinical functioning scores for each of these three groups. The meaning of each scale point can be approximated as follows: A score of 0, or "chronic," meant that, on average, the patient spent three-quarters of the follow-up period institutionalized and was virtually unemployed, socially isolated, and symptomatic the entire time. A score of 1, or "marginal," indicated that the patient was likely to spend about one-quarter of the follow-up period in sheltered settings, work about one-fifth of the time, experience some role-specific social contacts, and cope with symptomatic expressions of illness for about three-quarters of the period. A score of 2, or "moderate," meant that the patient spent a small amount of follow-up time in structured settings, worked more than half of the time, had friends but saw them infrequently, and experienced some time free of symptoms. A score of 3, or "good," indicated that the patient was seldom rehospitalized (and never for lengthy periods), was employed and socially active most of the time, and remained symptom free for the majority of the follow-up period. A score of 4, or "recovered," was similar to a score of 3, or "good," on these dimensions but indicated better function. Furthermore, recovered patients were usually capable of stable intimacy or generativity in relationships.

Figure 2–1 highlights the differences between the diagnostic groups, especially between schizophrenia group on the one hand and the unipolar affective disorder and BPD groups on the other. If a global score of 2 or more is taken as representing a reasonable outcome, only one-third of the schizophrenia patients reached such a state, compared with about three-fourths of the unipolar affective disorder patients and about four-fifths of the BPD patients. More unipolar affective disorder patients than BPD patients had chronically compromised functioning, but more also reached a state of complete recovery. A plurality of BPD patients were rated as having a good outcome, but lingering problems, mostly of a characterological nature, prevented them from achieving recovery more frequently.

When we focused on the BPD cohort, the following clinical profile emerged. Consistent with other studies of BPD clinical populations, the

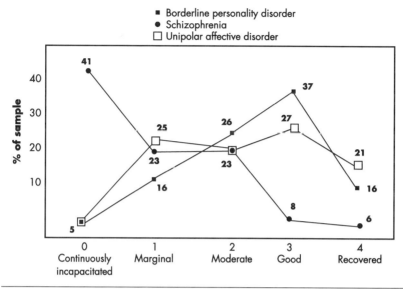

FIGURE 2–1. Frequency distribution of Clinical Global Functioning Scale scores since discharge for patients with borderline personality disorder and comparison groups.

majority of our BPD patients were single and female. Onset of disorder was usually in late adolescence, with illness escalating through the 20s. Onset was seldom precipitated by specific stress but appeared more in the nature of a pattern change in behavior to altered developmental demands. Before their first psychiatric contact, BPD patients were likely to have at least moderate impairment in all adaptive spheres—social, sexual, and instrumental. First treatment contact occurred in the 20s, as with the schizophrenia patients but not as with the unipolar affective disorder patients. Like most patients referred to Chestnut Lodge, the BPD cohort patients were chronically ill and had experienced many prior treatment experiences without remarkable success. For the BPD patients, however, prior treatment experiences were more likely to be in the form of outpatient psychosocial treatment than inpatient and somatic treatments, which were more usual for the schizophrenia patients. Also, in keeping with the classification of BPD as an Axis II personality disorder, our BPD patients were less ill at their index (Chestnut Lodge) admission in the nature and degree of manifest symptoms.

Although treated residentially without time limitations, the BPD patients at Chestnut Lodge did not tend to become institutionalized. Their inpatient time was the shortest of the diagnostic groups, and they were among the least likely to require transfer to other institutions. They were also far less passive and compliant—traits characteristic of the "institutionalized patient"—as evidenced by a high rate of signing out of the hospital against medical advice.

At follow-up, the BPD patients were doing well in their basic living situations. Most lived autonomously, some with intimate partners and some with children. They were similar to the unipolar affective disorder patients in this regard and were strikingly divergent from the schizophrenia patients.

Hospitalizations required by some of the BPD patients after Chestnut Lodge were frequently brief and crisis oriented. Although medication treatment, still in its infancy, was not used extensively after discharge, psychosocial outpatient treatments (usually individual or group psychotherapy) were very common, with nearly half of the patients requesting or requiring further therapeutic support.

Instrumentally, BPD patients proved quite productive in terms of both amount and quality of work, and they generally accumulated good work records. In fact, many appeared to work diligently despite an otherwise dismal existence. Also, BPD patients scored a mean of 2.9 on the Hollingshead scale of occupational level (Hollingshead and Redlich 1958) at follow-up, indicating jobs equivalent to administrative managers, small-business owners, minor professionals, and so on. This relatively high occupational level rating, compared with the other groups, may simply reflect good baseline socioeconomic status, but the BPD patients were able to make productive use of such resources.

As intense and unstable relationships are a key feature of the disorder, their outcome in this domain was of particular interest. At follow-up, the Chestnut Lodge BPD patients proved to be moderately active socially. On this dimension, however, the distribution of scores was bimodal. One major group had managed to create and maintain meaningful relationships with stability over time. This group further divided roughly into three subgroups: good social relationships but no intimate relationships; partial intimate relationships but no children; and intact intimate relationships with children. The other major group of patients, however, handled relationships by a studious avoidance of them and, in terms of the model presented in Chapter 1, appeared to employ a dismissing/detached form of attachment. They appeared to have concluded that it was not possible to maintain their emotional equilibrium in intimate relationships. On average, for the entire BPD group, relationships became less stormy and intense with time, but often the price was superficiality, avoidance, or isolation.

Most BPD patients demonstrated some evidence of persisting clinical symptoms that they often managed to compartmentalize and effectively prevent from interfering with their instrumental capacities. Depressive signs and symptoms were very common, as was substance abuse.

In summary, at follow-up, we found our patients with BPD doing quite well on the whole. Our findings were at variance with previous follow-up reports of adult borderline patients studied prior to the advent of DSM-III criteria (Carpenter and Gunderson 1977; Carpenter et al. 1977; Grinker et al. 1968; Gunderson et al. 1975; Pope et al. 1983; Werble 1970). Three long term follow-up studies (10–22 years) of DSM-III-diagnosed BPD patients were conducted contemporaneously with ours (Paris et al. 1987; Plakun et al. 1985; Stone et al. 1987). These findings basically replicated ours and strongly suggested that the thrust toward long-term improvement noted in our BPD patients was a robust finding and not unique to Chestnut Lodge's population. These findings have been further validated by several subsequent studies of the natural course and outcome of personality disorders (mostly BPD), reviewed elsewhere (Sanislow and McGlashan 1998).

BPD Profiles of Outcome by Sex and Follow-Up Length

We were interested in whether outcome varied with time after discharge. The outcome scores for the BPD patients varied significantly with time postdischarge. As illustrated in Figure 2–2, these patients' global outcome profile traced an inverted U, with the highest point occurring in the second postdischarge decade, when the average subject was in her or his 40s (McGlashan 1986).

We also found, on closer scrutiny, that male and female BPD patients differed in several aspects of their clinical profiles. This, and the variability in functioning over time, prompted an investigation into the long-term natural history of BPD by sex (Bardenstein and McGlashan 1988). We divided the follow-up period into three time intervals—0–9 years, 10–19 years, and 20+ years postdischarge—and compared BPD patients across follow-up interval and across sex.

The natural history of our residentially treated female BPD patient can be described as follows. Her premorbid and morbid functioning was characterized by multiple symptoms, especially depression and unstable marital/heterosexual relationships. In the first phase postdischarge, there was a continuation of these symptoms, often exacerbated by the loss of hospital structure and support. More severe symptomatic episodes seemed to be episodic, occasionally warranting further, but briefer, hospitalizations.

The woman with BPD, at least from this era, sought stability and need satisfaction in intimate relationships. She seemed capable of being

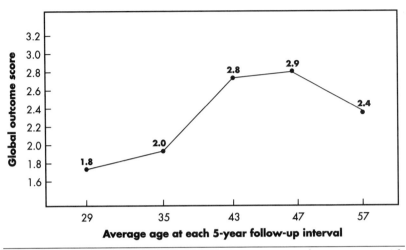

FIGURE 2–2. Global outcome, by follow-up age, for patients with borderline personality disorder.

productive so long as she had an intact and stable relationship. As she began to develop occupationally in the second decade postdischarge, hospitalization and outpatient treatment became less necessary. Her symptoms diminished in severity but could still be episodically severe. Prescription drugs for somatic complaints replaced self-medication with alcohol or illicit drugs.

With advancing age, the woman with BPD became more symptomatic again, especially if she lost her stable relationships through divorce or death. Although her instrumental competence continued to develop, her interpersonal contacts dwindled. Outpatient treatment and work were the predominant sources of stability, continuity, structure, and social contact.

Continued involvement in heterosexual relationships was present in most cases and appeared to play an important role in the woman's adjustment. In contrast to the woman with schizophrenia in the follow-up study, for whom marriage was associated with better socialization and occupational functioning (McGlashan and Bardenstein 1988), the woman with BPD who was married more often than not experienced an exacerbation of symptoms. Even though married, she frequently remained socially isolated, with superficial and infrequent contact with friends. Her great neediness appeared to preclude an ability to nurture or care for others, and she frequently had estranged relationships with her children.

The postdischarge profile of our residentially treated male BPD patients differed from that of our female BPD patients in both pattern and detail. The male BPD patient usually left the institution against medical advice (AMA). His initial period after discharge was characterized by continuing typical symptoms and trouble with the law. The male BPD patient maintained little contact with mental health professionals or institutions. He worked at various jobs somewhat nomadically. He remained single, lived alone, and socialized frequently but superficially. Major antisocial symptoms appeared to diminish in intensity, but not the avoidant pattern or lack of direction seen premorbidly.

The second phase after hospitalization included finding an occupational identity and achieving a stable income and sense of competency. Mild depression often continued, but the tendency toward avoidance was ameliorated by structured interpersonal contacts through work. The man with BPD clearly relied more on institutional than on intimate interpersonal relationships for gratification and structure.

In the third phase after hospitalization, the man with BPD consolidated and improved on his career and enjoyed the greater activity that ensued. He tolerated and even sought longer relationships and often considered marriage. He developed further support systems through other institutional affiliations, such as religious membership or participation in Alcoholics Anonymous. As described earlier for some of the female BPD patients, he developed a dismissing/detached form of attachment and could maintain closeness while remaining comfortably at a distance.

Methodological Limitations of the Follow-Up Study

Because of the cost of intensive long-term residential treatment provided at Chestnut Lodge, only those with means or unusual insurance policies could afford it. Thus, the reader will note that the patients presented are second- or third-generation inheritants of highly successful entrepreneurs. Although this results in a biased sample, we believe that their inherited wealth served both as a risk factor and as a protective factor in the course of the disorder. As the case histories illustrate, inherited wealth poses special problems and does not protect the individual from disorder or misery. It can, however, protect from extreme consequences such as homelessness and provide the opportunity for the best help available.

Since we lacked a control sample, we could not address the degree to which our findings reflected "normal" aging trends. Nevertheless, the sex-specific interactions of BPD pathology with time parallel observations of the general population from this historical time period (1950–1975); specifically, men relied more on work for satisfaction, whereas women relied more on relationships (Cleary and Mechanic 1983). The influence of such cultural parameters may have been critical given the era in which our sample lived. Around the middle of this century, women had less opportunity or encouragement to live independently and to develop careers. There was social pressure to get married and to be supported by the husband. This may account for much of the female BPD patient's more limited and vulnerable interpersonal adjustment.

We did not track changes across time in the same individual, nor did we use the same rating scales as repeated measures. The natural history profiles represent composites of individuals in different follow-up intervals rather than narratives of the same individual across follow-up intervals. As such, many of our results may stem from sample biasing, especially cohort effects. Furthermore, our male BPD patients may have been skewed toward better functioning because their more violent, alcoholic, antisocial, and criminal counterparts were incarcerated rather than hospitalized. While male and female BPD patients did not differ in severity of illness at admission, the possibility that the most seriously disturbed men with BPD were screened out at admission qualifies our findings.

SELECTION OF CASES FOR THE BOOK

The four cases presented here were the result of an intensive case-study process conducted by the coauthors. All case material for the 81 BPD patients identified for the follow-up study, available on microfiche and/or paper records in the Chestnut Lodge Medical Records Archives, was reviewed in preparation for this book. We selected the four cases of female BPD patients that best illustrated the characteristics of the disorder and its variability in course and outcome. The case material for the final four selected was drawn from all patient records available, including all therapist notes, nursing notes, records of occupational and art therapy activities, and transcriptions of case conferences; from follow-up interviews; and, when possible, from interviews with the original treating psychiatrist. Although we chose female patients, because women are more commonly seen in treatment for BPD than men, this work applies equally to male BPD patients.

In the next four chapters, we describe the case histories of these four Chestnut Lodge patients. The material is a condensation and integration of the voluminous records available and follows a standard case presentation format. At the end of each chapter, we discuss the etiology of the patient's disorder and the outcome according to the developmental model presented in Chapter 1. We conclude each chapter with a discussion of the patient's treatment.

REFERENCES

American Psychiatric Association: Diagnostic and Statistical Manual: Mental Disorders. Washington, DC, American Psychiatric Association, 1952

American Psychiatric Association: Diagnostic and Statistical Manual of Mental Disorders, 2nd Edition. Washington, DC, American Psychiatric Association, 1968

Bardenstein KK, McGlashan TH: The natural history of a residentially treated borderline sample: gender differences. Journal of Personality Disorders 2:69–83, 1988

Carpenter WT, Gunderson JG: Five year follow-up comparison of borderline and schizophrenic patients. Compr Psychiatry 18:567–571, 1977

Carpenter WT, Gunderson JG, Strauss JS: Considerations of the borderline syndrome: a longitudinal comparative study of borderline and schizophrenic patients, in Borderline Personality Disorders: The Concept, the Syndrome, the Patient. Edited by Hartocollis P. New York, International Universities Press, 1977, pp 223–254

Cleary PH, Mechanic D: Sex differences in psychological distress among married people. J Health Soc Behav 24:111–121, 1983

Fromm-Reichmann F: Principles of Intensive Psychotherapy (1950). Chicago, IL, University of Chicago Press, 1960

Grinker R, Werble B, Drye R: The Borderline Syndrome: A Behavioral Study of Ego Functions. New York, Basic Books, 1968

Gunderson JG, Kolb JE: Discriminating features of borderline patients. Am J Psychiatry 135:792–796, 1978

Gunderson JG, Carpenter WT, Strauss J: Borderline and schizophrenic patients: a comparative study. Am J Psychiatry 132:1257–1264, 1975

Hollingshead AB, Redlich FC: Social Class and Mental Illness. New York, Wiley, 1958

McGlashan TH: The Chestnut Lodge Follow-Up Study, Part I: follow-up methodology and study sample. Arch Gen Psychiatry 41:573–585, 1984a

McGlashan TH: The Chestnut Lodge Follow-Up Study, Part II: long-term outcome of schizophrenia and affective disorders. Arch Gen Psychiatry 41: 586–601, 1984b

McGlashan T: The Chestnut Lodge Follow-Up Study, Part III: long-term outcome of borderline personalities. Arch Gen Psychiatry 42:20–30, 1986

McGlashan TH: The longitudinal profile of borderline personality disorder: contributions from the Chestnut Lodge Follow-Up Study, in Handbook of Borderline Disorders. Edited by Silver D, Rosenbluth M. New York, International Universities Press, 1992, pp 53–83

McGlashan TH, Bardenstein KK: Schizotypal personality disorder: gender differences. Journal of Personality Disorders 2:221–227, 1988

Paris J, Brown R, Nowlis D: Long-term follow-up of borderline patients in a general hospital. Compr Psychiatry 28:530–535, 1987

Plakun EM, Burkhardt PE, Muller JP: Fourteen year follow-up of borderline schizotypal personality disorders. Compr Psychiatry 26:448–455, 1985

Pope HG Jr, Jonas JM, Hudson JI, et al: The validity of the DSM-III borderline personality disorder. Arch Gen Psychiatry 40:23–30, 1983

Sanislow CA, McGlashan TH: Treatment outcome of personality disorders. Can J Psychiatry 43:237–250, 1998

Stone MH, Hurt SW, Stone DK: The P.I.-500: long-term follow-up of borderline in-patients meeting DSM-III criteria, I: global outcome. Journal of Personality Disorders 1:291–298, 1987

Werble B: Second follow-up study of borderline patients. Arch Gen Psychiatry 23: 3–7, 1970

3

When She Was Good…Lillian

When she was good
She was very, very good
And when she was bad
She was horrid

Nursery rhyme

Lillian Rand, labeled the "Bad Seed" by her parents, presented to staff at Chestnut Lodge with signs typical of BPD: identity diffusion, substance abuse, promiscuity, and dissociation. She eagerly entered Chestnut Lodge at the age of 20, fearing that she was about to "crack, fall into dust and blow away." For 2 weeks prior to her admission, she haunted the bars near her home and in alcoholic stupors took one man after another home to bed in a desperate attempt to fill the emptiness left after giving up her newborn daughter for adoption.

HISTORY OF DISORDER

Lillian's mother first took her for psychiatric consultation at the age of 6, concerned about her withdrawn and detached behavior and her inability to read. At age 11, Lillian went on rampages in the house while in a "zombie-like" state during her mother's hospitalization for an illness, and another psychiatric consultation was arranged. Tutorial help in reading was given but not treatment. Also, a binge-eating disorder without obesity was evident by the age of 11. During the seventh grade, Lillian found that sexual involvement brought her back from feeling "far away." From this point on she engaged in promiscuous sexual relationships. Her choice of partners was boys from the "acting-out elements" in school and community who were also within her social class. Lillian lived a dual life, participating in extracurricular activities and developing artistic abilities while secretly engaging in sexual liaisons and substance abuse.

The strain of her double life led to increased depression, withdrawal, and detachment. Alarmed by her falling grades, her mother consulted a psychiatrist. With the help of psychotherapy for her emotional problems and remedial help for her long-standing reading disability, Lillian maintained active involvement in school committees and plays and graduated from high school.

After graduation, Lillian applied for admission to an art school and was accepted. She expressed great relief to be leaving home, but the family tumult continued long distance, as she was on the phone regularly, nagging and badgering her parents for more money and clothes. Lillian did well in the art courses, and one of her pieces was chosen for exhibit. However, her academic course work suffered as her reading disability continued.

She continued to engage in brief sexual relationships, but she now taunted her parents openly with her exploits. Alarmed by her blatant and blasé talk of sex and her poor grades, Lillian's parents enlisted her former psychiatrist's help, and Lillian returned to see him during the summer vacation. After this, she struggled through another year but ultimately decided to leave school and move to another city where she had friends.

Now 19 years old, Lillian was unable to cope in the new city. She came home to live with her parents and returned to treatment. She rapidly found home "intolerable"; took a sales job, where she was well accepted; and set up her own apartment. She continued to engage in brief but intense sexual liaisons. However, for the first time she met a young man who seemed to be invested in her personally and fell wildly in love with him. After their first sexual contact, she became pregnant. Initially, she considered marrying him, but she soon devalued the relationship and described him as a "wasted pathetic character." She did not tell him of the pregnancy for 4 months, and when he offered to marry her, she refused.

Lillian never considered abortion, which was illegal at the time and difficult to obtain. She remained silent about her pregnancy except to her psychiatrist and on her own made arrangements with an adoption agency to assist her with the birth and placement of her child. During the pregnancy, Lillian stayed in her apartment and continued working.

Lillian's parents later expressed astonishment at her deceit. They visited periodically but suspected nothing.

Lillian gave her child up for adoption without seeing her, fearing she would become attached. She "cried a great deal" after the delivery and wished the situation were different. She expressed relief that the child would not be raised as she had been. During the postpartum weeks, her psychiatrist noted that she "pulled herself together, kept her apartment clean, and talked in terms of positive self-concept and values." However, this lasted only briefly. She became increasingly depressed, drank heavily, and engaged in sexual relations with a variety of men.

When her mother stopped by Lillian's apartment unannounced one day, she found Lillian in bed with yet another man. An argument ensued, and Lillian blurted out, "I had a bastard child this summer. Don't tell Daddy or he'll have a heart attack." Mother called Lillian's psychiatrist and expressed hopelessness over the course of Lillian's life. He, too, was alarmed by her erratic behavior and noted she was missing more and more appointments with him. Feeling disruption in the therapeutic alliance and concern that Lillian might harm herself, he recommended hospitalization at Chestnut Lodge, and Lillian readily agreed.

FAMILY HISTORY

In Lillian's parents and grandparents there is evidence for anxiety and depressive disorders, alcoholism, and histrionic and narcissistic (Cluster B) personality traits. Both grandfathers were highly successful but difficult men. One grandmother, a fiery redhead, was known as the "holy terror." The other was a prominent socialite who was intensely critical and intolerant of bad manners. This grandmother locked Lillian's mother in a closet for minor transgressions and would not speak to her for days on end during her childhood.

Lillian's father was supported by a family trust, and he invested in one failed venture after another. He referred to himself as a sales executive but maintained a "pseudo" office. Most of his time was spent hunting and fishing, at which he found greater success. Mr. Rand suffered from episodic depressions complicated by alcoholism. When Mr. Rand was drunk, his usually self-deprecating demeanor was transformed, and he erupted into tirades against his wife and engaged in screaming matches with Lillian, who became his nemesis. He was in psychoanalysis throughout most of Lillian's youth.

Lillian's mother was also a prominent socialite. Mrs. Rand was described as a charming and intelligent woman with "peaches and cream" complexion who made a point of how pretty she looked. Lillian criticized her mother for being a "status seeker" and superficial. Mrs. Rand was a highly competent organizer and fund-raiser and sat on the boards of many civic and charitable organizations. She developed panic attacks and depressive symptoms during both of her pregnancies, as had her mother before her. She engaged in intensive brief psychotherapy after Lillian's birth and maintained a supportive relationship with this psychiatrist throughout her life.

Lillian's only sibling was her sister Kate, 2 years younger. Kate resembled her mother in temperament and appearance, whereas Lillian was similar to her father. Kate was the "good girl" who "saved her money and was pure and chaste" and a model of decorum. Although Kate described herself during the hospital interviews as a "happy, normal teenager," she had several bouts of depression after entering college that eventually lead to treatment.

DEVELOPMENTAL HISTORY

Lillian was born within the first year of her parent's marriage, and Mr. Rand designated her birth as the beginning of unending trouble in the family. Mrs. Rand did not enjoy her pregnancy. Her preoccupation with weight caused her to hold in her stomach, and she experienced considerable anxiety. Labor was prolonged and painful because "Lillian's head was too big." Mrs. Rand was frightened of her newborn, and Mr. Rand experienced intensely jealous feelings of being displaced.

Mrs. Rand, although advised not to, nursed Lillian despite extreme physical pain caused by split nipples. Lillian nursed frantically for a few minutes and then fell asleep. Mrs. Rand felt unable to satisfy her, a theme that continued throughout their relationship. Lillian walked by 10 months, suggesting precocious motor development. She was described as a bright, responsive, and strong-willed child who smiled all of the time.

Lillian's family was plagued by illness during her early years. When Lillian was 8 months old, Mrs. Rand was hospitalized for exploratory surgery. At 18 months, Mr. Rand was hospitalized with tuberculosis. Lillian had a recurring, vivid memory of being forbidden to touch or be anywhere near her father. Six months after father was quarantined with TB, mother gave birth to Kate and Lillian went to live with her paternal grandparents. After Kate's birth it was discovered that the paternal grandmother had a debilitating illness. At age 3, Lillian suffered from life-threatening pneumonia, and Kate was diagnosed with a chronic metabolic illness. Mrs. Rand hired a live-in nurse for Kate, and Lillian's care was delegated to the housekeeper. Mrs. Rand was up nightly with Kate and had few resources left during the day for Lillian.

Family life was unhappy and tumultuous. Lillian and her father engaged in frequent verbal fights, each one trying to get in the last word. Lillian resorted to temper tantrums and was a "nagger and whiner" when she didn't get her way. When her father drank, he became verbally abusive to her mother, who would cry helplessly.

At 8 months, Lillian exhibited "zombie-states" during which she would seem detached and "far away." Although toilet trained at the usual time of development, Lillian developed a habit of "willfully" having bowel movements in the middle of the floor or in closets during periods of separation from her parents. By the age 4, Lillian displayed fierce temper tantrums, at which times she would throw and smash objects in the house. Her recall of this early childhood period was of feeling unprotected and neglected.

By the age 6, Lillian felt dissociated much of the time, appeared withdrawn, and, in her first year of school, was unable to learn how to read. In response to Lillian's reading problem and withdrawal, Mrs. Rand had her evaluated by a child psychoanalyst. In the 1960s there was minimal awareness of learning disabilities, and most school problems were viewed as a sign of laziness or psychological problems. It is unknown what kind of assessment was conducted, but the family was reassured that Lillian had good mental abilities and did not require further treatment. Still, Lillian struggled with reading and, as a result, was a mediocre student.

COURSE IN TREATMENT AT HOME AND AT CHESTNUT LODGE

Lillian had her first psychotherapy experience in high school, and a summary of treatment was available in the records. Her psychiatrist, Dr. Richards, appeared genuinely interested in Lillian's welfare and saw her as someone with "considerable talent" and "sincerely interested in treatment. "In his referral letter to Chestnut Lodge, he exhorted staff not to be taken in by Lillian's facade of "self-sufficiency" but to see a frightened girl underneath who fears rejection. He urged the new doctor to communicate a "direct, straightforward interest." His diagnosis was of a "severe depression" that was covered over by her "differences with her parents."

The early course of the relationship was characterized by Lillian "testing" whether Dr. Richards "considered her a worthwhile person" and provoking him in many ways until she "settled on sexual acting-out." Dr. Richards described himself as "very active . . . [alternating] among support, strong confrontation, and direct interpretation . . . to handle the acting out." He believed that therapy helped her to graduate from high school and to apply to art school. He encouraged her decision to leave home so that she could disengage from the family battles.

Lillian left school, returned home, and returned to treatment with Dr. Richards. He was alarmed over her sexual behavior and drinking and considered "sanitarium care" as a form of "protection" for her. Ulti-mately, they agreed to four times weekly outpatient psychotherapy. De-spite this, Lillian's behavior continued to veer out of control, and Dr. Richards felt ineffective. His decision to refer Lillian for residential care was in response to pressure from Mrs. Rand and his feeling that outpa-tient therapy could not provide sufficient containment.

In the Chestnut Lodge admission note, Lillian, 20, was described as bright, artistic, and attractive. Her "language was quite coarse" but she was open and appeared to want to confide in someone. The dissociative quality immediately impressed staff, as they noted that although Lillian was verbal, she was very detached and "told her story without much feeling." The admissions doctor rated his personal feelings toward Lil-lian as "strongly attracted." It is interesting that his initial diagnosis was schizoid personality, probably related to Lillian's dissociative, detached style.

During the initial family meeting, the social worker noted that Lillian was the spokesperson for the family in that she was able to "say things out in the open . . . easily." She was the only one in the family who really said what she wanted. She swore a lot and insulted her parents, while they appeared, the social worker noted, "phony and talked on the top of things" and actually referred to themselves as a "phony bunch." When Lillian left the initial family session, the parents criticized her insulting behavior and stated that any trouble the family ever had was related to her, beginning with Mrs. Rand's pregnancy. They called her a "con artist" and manipulator. However, during the session they accepted her insults silently and appeared to admire and envy her honesty.

Mrs. Rand wrote letters to the social worker on a regular basis, pro-viding additional information on Lillian interspersed with comments about herself and her husband. There is an effusive, dramatic quality to these letters, with frequent use of exclamation points. The parents phoned Lillian several times weekly and visited the hospital every 6 weeks. It was the staff's impression that Mr. Rand seemed to tag along and allow his wife to take the lead. In family sessions, he appeared to feel inade-quate and troubled.

As part of the admission process, psychological testing was administered routinely. On the Wechsler Adult Intelligence Scale, Lillian demonstrated superior functioning in her nonverbal abilities, with a Performance IQ of 137. Her verbal abilities were in the above-average range, with a Verbal IQ of 119. The 18-point difference between Lillian's verbal and performance abilities is not unusual for individuals with high intelligence. However, the direction of the difference supports the existence of the reported reading disability. The hospital psychologist noted that Lillian did not "reflect or concentrate on a verbally formulated problem but could perform quickly and accurately . . . when the problem is nonverbal." Her superior visuospatial abilities expressed themselves in her artistic abilities.

The Rorschach descriptions reflect Lillian's problems in cognitive integration of her interpersonal world. To her the blots reflected a nihilistic view of the world in which everything is "ugly, unreal, meaningless, unconnected chaos!" She was unable to elaborate on concepts but gave only quick impressions. Relationships were seen as either symbiotically close and structuring or completely undependable and disconnected. As this evaluation was conducted before the advent of the DSM-III diagnosis of BPD, the psychologist made a tentative diagnosis of personality trait disturbance with schizoid, depressive, and antisocial features.

Lillian was assigned to Dr. Davis, a medical staff psychiatrist, who saw her for psychoanalytic psychotherapy four times weekly until he was drafted into the army 6 months later. When asked during the initial case conference how he felt toward her, he said, "I like her; I like her very much!" He was impressed with her desire to talk and noted that he had a hard time "cutting her off." He also noted that although she talked a great deal, she did not provide much "data." He found Lillian's reasoning hard to follow; her verbalizations lacked detail and integration. She expressed a wish to have her "head screwed on right" and referred to feeling "nutsy and squirrely" prior to admission. Her language was vague and imprecise; when asked how she was feeling, she usually said, "Nervous." In alluding to her dissociative states she often complained of going "blank" and not being able to hear what others were saying to her. Her difficulty integrating experience or "putting things together in a sensible way" and "glossing over of emotions" became a major focus of the therapy.

During the first few weeks of the therapy, Lillian talked about her pregnancy and baby. She brought letters into the sessions that she had received from her mother and friends. She often brought Cracker Jacks to share and liked to bring in her recent paintings for Dr. Davis's admiration. Dr. Davis was struck by her inability to talk about what was going on in her life, and the letters and art appeared to provide a medium for communication. During this early stage, Lillian conveyed a wish to marry an Al Hurt/Burl Ives/Santa Claus type of man with a lot of money. The image of a warm, folksy fatherly figure provides a glimpse into Lillian's need for a nurturant parent and how she had transferred that need onto men.

Lillian displayed considerable identity confusion during her sessions. One day she would have her hair up, one day down; one day she would wear heels, the next day Japanese sandals. She sat in one session with considerable thigh exposed, another with slouched masculine nonchalance, and another with feet primly beneath her. Dr. Davis described Lillian coming to one session with her hair in a French knot, dressed in high heels with black stockings and popping bubble gum throughout the session.

Lillian was especially concerned that Dr. Davis be "himself" and react to her in a genuine and honest fashion. She criticized her former therapist for being a "phony." Her parents had described themselves as a "phony bunch," referring to their inability to be direct about their feelings and the disparity between their successful social persona and contrasting family conflict. In Lillian's home, straightforward communication was rare. She styled herself as a truth sayer and needed the same from her therapist.

Lillian gradually developed an ability to talk about the details of her daily activities in the hospital. For the first time, she exhibited an improvement in the integration of affect and thought. When she looked unhappy, she was able to say she felt miserable and had fleeting suicidal thoughts.

Unlike many patients with BPD, Lillian did not exhibit any dramatic self-destructive behaviors such as self-mutilation, either before or during her hospitalization. The only "acting out" incident occurred during the first weeks of her hospitalization and was minor. Lillian left the grounds without permission and met with a former male aide. Also around this same time, she and a male patient were seen "pinching each other in embarrassing places." Other than these minor incidents, she was described as a model patient who adjusted quickly to the ward. Lillian appeared hungry for routine and clear structure.

Lillian developed a close relationship with a female patient and preferred spending time with her rather than at hospital activities. The only activities in which she did engage were group art projects. Staff felt she was "extremely creative" but lacked discipline; she would quit if the job could not be completed at one sitting. She also displayed a demeaning attitude toward others whom she did not respect and could be impatient and critical of their creative efforts.

Lillian soon developed a romantic relationship with a male patient, Michael. Dr. Johnson, watching Lillian and Michael walk by his office window, observed Lillian following 20 paces behind the rapidly pacing Michael. At first Dr. Johnson thought Lillian was pursuing Michael, then being dragged after him. His final impression was one of an Indian with his squaw.

Three months into the therapy Dr. Davis announced that he had been drafted. Lillian became frightened and disoriented. Dr. Davis regretted leaving. He interpreted the transference as Lillian acting toward him as an "idealized older brother whom she often imagined having while growing up." This idealization quickly reversed around the time of Dr. Davis's departure. In their last session, Lillian's disappointment in Dr. Davis was transformed into a demeaning and critical stance. She informed him that she suspected he was stupid at their first meeting and allowing himself to be drafted confirmed her suspicions.

In the initial hospitalwide case conference regarding Lillian's care, Dr. Davis presented his work with her. There was considerable discussion of Lillian's dissociation and depersonalization. Lillian had dissociated throughout her life and appeared unperturbed by things to which she should have reacted. The staff speculated that Lillian employed massive denial and as a result lived in a different reality or had lived with two realities at once. Indeed, there appeared to be two Lillian's: one who was competent and social, interacting with mischievous humor and talent, and the other who was detached, withdrawn, and given to solipsistic behaviors. Her sexual behavior appeared to be a bridge between her two selves, a means to restore contact with the human world and feelings.

The participants in this first case conference were struggling to "know" Lillian and found it difficult. There was much discussion regarding whether to contact her former therapist and how much involvement there should be with the family. Many felt that the previous therapist had been too involved with the family. Everyone worried about boundaries and moves from overinvolvement to distance and neglect, thus enacting the disorganized relatedness schemas of Lillian's earlier experiences.

After Dr. Davis's departure, Lillian was transferred to Dr. Peters, whom she saw over the next 15 months as an inpatient. Dr. Peters' initial impression of Lillian was that she was "eager to talk, childish, scattered and anxious." She angrily railed against the incompetence of psychiatrists and of those who tried to coerce her into a conventional mold. He also found her "extremely, infectiously amusing."

Within a few weeks of their first meeting, she idealized Dr. Peters, expressing how strong and good he was and how she felt she could lean on him. Alongside this idealization Dr. Peters detected a parallel mocking contempt and disgust with psychiatry that he believed covered a feeling of being assaulted by therapy. There were also "hints at a sexual preoccupation" with him. Concurrent with her new therapeutic relationships, Lillian became intensely involved with another male patient, Robert. The hospital staff and Dr. Peters commented on her slavish devotion to him. Lillian, insulted by this allegation, vehemently denied it and asserted that she was the one with power and control, not Robert.

In the medical staff case conference, Dr. Peters provided detailed descriptions of several characteristic response patterns in the psychotherapy that occurred early on and became thematic. Two months into treatment she began to ask for discharge from the hospital. He told her that she would first have to find an apartment and a job. Lillian proceeded to make "monotonous, repetitive, painful demands to be let go." During one of these sessions, in which she was especially "childish, whiny, and demanding," Dr. Peters confronted her whining. Lillian experienced the confrontation as a threat to the relationship. She appeared stunned; her speech became rapid and pressured, and her baby talk became more pronounced. Dr. Peters felt shut out by her rapid speech and again confronted her, stating she did not want to hear what he had to say. She appeared hurt and depressed and told him she felt discouraged and confused and that she was shattering inside and flying to pieces. She reported intrusive images of breaking windows. This was followed by expressed wishes to sit with him and to put her head on his lap and cry. Lillian expressed a fear that he would leave her and told him how much she depended on him, pleading that he tolerate and stay with her. He experienced vague feelings of being seduced during this exchange.

During another session she listed all of the people she had manipulated and demeaned, including the men with whom she had slept. Dr. Peters confronted the latter, speculating that she had been the one exploited. The suggestion that she was the one who was the victim assaulted her grandiose sense of self. Stunned and bewildered, she stated, "I feel screwy," suggesting a return of depersonalization. She then dug her nails into her hands until it hurt, a self-mutilation equivalent, to prove to him how much control she had over painful feelings. Now she wanted to go out and "turn someone into mush."

Within the first few months of their relationship Lillian had clearly developed an intense attachment to Dr. Peters. She complained of feeling controlled by him, of losing herself and fading away, yet she requested more of his time. She wanted Dr. Peters to love her and for them to have a special private language. She longed for him to be able to read her mind and had images of them being twins with brains attached. During some sessions she would gaze at him with devotion and at other times with "sultry lingering and dramatic looks." When she realized that Dr. Peters could not read her mind, she felt lonely and developed headaches. Around Dr. Peters's August vacation, Lillian expressed a concern that she would be lost and might die without him. She feared that on his return he would stop working with her unless she gave up her relationship with Robert and lived as a nun. She accused him of being jealous of this relationship and of trying to take the fun out of her life. She needed Robert because Dr. Peters could only see her 1 hour a day.

The anniversary of her daughter's adoption occurred at this juncture, and Lillian expressed a wish that Dr. Peters's could have been the father, confident that he would have been a good father. She expressed jealousy of his children and became as disoriented as when she signed the adoption papers. In a dream, Lillian looked into Dr. Peters's office and saw him teaching his beautiful golden-haired daughter about life while using up Lillian's appointment time.

In September, after Dr. Peters' vacation, Lillian began looking for a job, and, concurrently, Robert was discharged from the hospital. She soon developed a fear that she was trapped in the hospital and Dr. Peters was going to rape her. This was accompanied by vivid fantasies of herself as a child alone with her father, locked in her room, believing that Farmer MacGregor, a storybook character, was coming to kill her. Disorganized, desperate, and intensely dysphoric, Lillian cried and begged Dr. Peters to stop the hurting feeling and to make her feel better. Without Robert, Lillian felt doomed by longings toward Dr. Peters and feared that nothing could fill the deep, empty gap revealed through the therapeutic relationship. She asked Dr. Peters to tell her stories like her father used to and again asked him to love her. At this point, however, she also expressed the fear that if he did love her it would be terrifying, as she would then be too powerful.

The following soliloquy which Dr. Peters wrote verbatim from a session during this period highlights Lillian's mental state:

> I feel weird . . . just goofy. I'm crazy . . . I'm raving mad. . . . I'm depressed. I keep thinking I'm going to drive a car into a tree. I'm going to drive it into a telephone pole and smash it up. It takes a lot of restraint not to do it. I didn't want to come today, I almost forgot. I've been eating like a pig all day and I didn't even take my contraceptive pill today. I don't want to be here at all. Can I go home? I keep getting these urges to do strange things. I had the thought of wanting to stop in the middle of Beechwood Avenue at heavy traffic and pick tulips in a garden. I want to sleep with you and my father and I can't do that either. I feel like cry-

ing again. All of a sudden I feel I should cry. I can't concentrate on anything. I would like to die. I don't like being unhappy. If I'm going to be unhappy, I should just die. I want to eliminate you from my life also. I don't want anyone around. Then I could be really miserable. I'd like to drive a horse with wings or a car 200 miles an hour. I can't do any of these things so I guess I'm asleep.

She ended the hour by reciting "Humpty-Dumpty," fearing she could never be put back together again. Dr. Peters saw her for extra sessions during these months and accepted phone calls when she was agitated and suicidal.

This intense period in the therapy was followed by Lillian's renewed campaign for discharge from the hospital. Instead of pleading with him to love and care for her completely, she now pled to be let go, and she barraged him with criticisms. Hour after hour, and repetitively within the hour, Lillian would cry, "Let me go, you're killing me." She compared "driving Dr. Peters to distraction" to similar interactions with her father. She recalled an incident when she and her Dad argued for hours over the birthplace of Ben Franklin. Even when mother found the answer in the encyclopedia, they continued to argue.

Dr. Peters began to feel increasingly inadequate in response to her demands and criticisms. He felt "self-disgust" and wondered if he were being "rigid and arbitrary." He communicated these feelings directly to her. She continued to express the full range of her feelings toward him with brutal honesty and directness.

Midway through the hospitalization Lillian visited home. She managed to stay out of most of her parent's arguments but could not resist making "annoying," deep interpretations of her Dad's behavior. Overall, however, she had a successful visit.

When she returned, Lillian focused on concerns about her feminine identity. She expressed fear of being a grown-up, sexual woman and described her former relationship with Robert as like "two little kids." She continued to look for work and began a new art project.

Over the next few months she continued her demands for release, but in a less punishing manner. Dr. Peters noted, "She managed to get some actual charm into it[,] which takes the edge off for me." At the same time, Lillian was actively looking for an appropriate job and thinking of courses she might take.

One year into treatment, Lillian began a part-time job in a museum. She felt valued and enjoyed her work. Dr. Peters felt a "great relief" that she had found something she enjoyed. This was accompanied by a cessation in Lillian's demands to be an outpatient as she now assumed it was forthcoming.

Lillian continued her attempts to determine where she stood with Dr. Peters and to learn the boundaries of the relationship. She threatened suicide to see if she could get a rise out of him. Her nagging insistence that he give her what she wanted was a deeply ingrained, interpersonal pattern that she described as "eroding you like water running down a rock." Although still enacting this behavior in therapy, Lillian was now able to observe herself. She referred to this behavior as "insane." She asked, "Why am I such a horrible kid?" and referred to herself as the "Bad Seed." She also became more aware of how her persistent nagging fights with her father were an attempt to get his attention and love. Lillian described how he never paid "true" attention to her except only as it affected him.

When her job became full-time and she found an apartment, Lillian anticipated missing the hospital, which no longer seemed a trap. Now she was concerned about being lonely. She readily accepted very early therapy hours to Dr. Peters's surprise after refusing them for some months. When she began spending nights out of the hospital, Lillian experienced disorganization in the sessions, fearing that Dr. Peters would lose interest in her as an outpatient.

Robert visited her for a few days at this time, and she asked him to shorten his visit in order to please Dr. Peters. Having done so, Lillian began a "blitz" to transition from outpatient to the status of a private patient. The standard progression at Chestnut Lodge was from inpatient to outpatient to private patient status. Lillian felt she had earned this change in status, but Dr. Peters felt it was precipitous. He experienced maintaining this limit as more "painful" than her previous campaigns to "go," as Lillian's success in the community made him feel less justified in keeping her connected to the hospital. He felt "ridiculous and arbitrary" in maintaining this limit, yet did so out of a conviction that the limit and the "hold" were important to her ultimate success at individuation.

As Dr. Peters adhered to his stance, Lillian initiated an "insistent grinding demand" that he tell her more about himself. His continued silence on this point escalated her frustration, and Lillian questioned whether she could trust him. Fantasies of sexual involvement with Dr. Peters reoccurred. She began to think of him as "mysterious, mystical, and unknowable" and wondered if she could continue working with him. These sexualized feelings triggered further associations to her father. She recalled fears of being touched by father, which earlier in her life were so severe that she was unable to shake hands with anyone. It is again unclear if this was a sign of early sexual abuse or related to her father's tuberculosis and the prohibition against touching him or being near him for 2 years. Lillian could only report that she experienced father as a frightening stranger. Her attempts to "know" Dr. Peters appeared to be a reenactment of trying to know and establish a satisfying relationship with her father substitute.

Dr. Peters noted that he avoided trying to "provide things other people didn't provide." He described what he did as "enduring my feelings and hers day after day" and focusing on what was going on in the here and now between the two of them. He unrelentingly focused on how she interpreted his verbal and nonverbal behavior. Dr. Peters had many concerns about his work with Lillian. He felt that his presentation in the medical staff case conferences would reveal him as "stuffy, rigid, conventional, and possibly inept." He saw his countertransference as a major problem.

During the last staff conference regarding Lillian's treatment, the important features of work were addressed. Some felt that Dr. Peters had provided a corrective experience in that no one in Lillian's life had persisted at the cost of so much fatigue and anxiety and with "such restraint and careful attention in helping her to differentiate her thoughts and behaviors so that the integrity of herself could be increased." Dr. Peters' feelings were likened to those of the mother of a young child who at the end of the day feels drained and empty.

Despite his concerns about his work, Dr. Peters made it clear that he felt hopeful about being able to endure with Lillian. When others worried that he might be giving up, he commented, "She takes very good care of me." He went on to explain that she "saves me from too much grief" by her sense of humor. When her scathing attacks and demands are on the brink of defeating him, she will suddenly make a funny comment and they will laugh. The relationship will be repaired, and they carry on. It was felt these comments captured the strength of the alliance as well as Lillian's capacity for growth and development.

Lillian was discharged to private-patient status after 18 months in the hospital and remained a private patient of Dr. Peters for one more year. At the time of discharge she was working in the community and settled in her own apartment and had established a network of local friends.

FOLLOW-UP TWELVE YEARS LATER

At follow-up, Lillian was in her mid 30s, had been married for the past 10 years, and lived with her husband in their home in an affluent suburb of a major metropolitan area. She worked as an executive in the fashion industry. Throughout the interview she engaged with the interviewer in an open and witty manner. She made frequent wry comments about others, and, as Dr. Peters had noted, her humor was infectious. She generated an aura of the busy highly pressured executive as she put the interviewer on frequent hold to answer business calls. She bantered with her husband in the background.

After discharge, Lillian saw Dr. Peters five times weekly for 6 months and then twice weekly until her termination 4 months later. She sought no further treatment during the 12-year follow-up period.

After terminating treatment, Lillian traveled in Europe for a few months and then returned to her hometown. After settling in, she accepted a job with a family friend. During this time she met her husband-to-be, Andrew, and through him became involved in the world of fashion. She and Andrew met in May and married in July.

Lillian felt this was more his choice than hers as "[i]t wasn't something that I felt a great need to do." She had trouble adjusting to the commitment of marriage and especially to sexual fidelity. The couple tried to set up rules for each other regarding involvement with others, but both became hurt in the process. They resolved to have an open marriage, believing that "emotional fidelity is more important than sexual fidelity."

During the first half of their marriage, when her husband was on extended business trips, Lillian said, "I would get seductive and carry on with anybody I was in the mood for. . . . I ended up sleeping with most of my men friends off and on." At the time of the follow-up interview, Lillian had not been involved with anyone in a "long, long time" and attributed this to her increased involvement with work, not to a change in attitude. Lillian had become pregnant twice and had had abortions each time during the earlier years of her marriage. She stated adamantly that she had never wanted children and that she "made fashion shows, not babies."

Lillian was proud and somewhat surprised by the solidity and length of her marriage. She noted blissful times and times when "you wish you weren't there." She expressed gratitude toward Andrew for "putting up with me all of these years," alluding to her early struggles around being married. Conflicts still arose around "who was smarter and who got the last word," reminiscent of her battles with her father, but she was better at letting it drop, and they would "go to a movie." Andrew was not always as supportive as she wished, but she acknowledged that neither was she.

Lillian said she rarely was sad or cried. The only time she remembered feeling upset was during a reunion with the father of the daughter she relinquished for adoption. She described him as "the only man in my life that ever made me . . . feel . . . in love and your stomach hurts and you're never quite happy . . . you've got 20 seconds of bliss and a lot of craziness." She reexperienced these emotions on seeing him and within a day withdrew, stating that she could not handle the "high drama."

A turning point in Lillian's life was leaving her hometown and moving to her current location. The couple bought their first home when she was promoted at work. Since the move, Lillian discovered she could assume greater work responsibility and conduct her life in a more disciplined and consistent manner. She managed to maintain her weight within a 5-pound instead of 30-pound range. She had far fewer "raging periods"—that is, times when she felt unhappy or frustrated and became a "TV junkie," smoked marijuana, or slept with her male friends. She attributed much of her improvement to the move and a change in diet.

In her leisure time, Lillian studied astrology, cooked, made crafts, and had recently designed an addition to their home. She saw friends regularly and considered herself to have "lots of close friends who are interactively supportive . . . someone you share things with . . . that you have mutual reliance . . . [and] enjoy the same interests." She felt more able to choose and reach out to friends who could provide support for specific needs. Lillian placed a high premium on intelligence and indicated that she did not suffer fools silently or for long.

Lillian saw herself as very self-sufficient and independent. While acknowledging that she relied on Andrew, she countered that this was due to habit and commented, "I could live without it." With friends and with Andrew she described an inability to tolerate "wallowing" in any emotion for too long. Similarly, she stated that if a relationship did not fulfill what she wanted or needed, she opted out quickly, stating, "I haven't got the patience to indulge them." However, she also maintained troubled relationships with some people over long periods of time. For example, Lillian tolerated a grade-school friend whom both her mother and husband disliked because she criticized Lillian to others often. Yet Lillian ignored such "unpleasant" aspects of their relationship and disengaged only after the woman accused her falsely of theft. Similarly, she tolerated her husband's "morose moods," perhaps unnecessarily. Lillian described herself as selfish, abrasive, combative without guilt, rarely sad, lucky, in control, confident, and competent. She joked that "if I don't get more humble at work, I'm in a lot of trouble."

Lillian's family members had undergone significant changes during the follow-up period. Her father had acknowledged his alcoholism after a serious medical complication and stopped drinking. Shortly afterward, he and Lillian's mother effected a stable separation. Lillian continued to see her father as a "schmuck" whom she did not like very much. Now, however, there was more kindness and civility than hostility between them. Lily saw her mother as a "terrific lady" and described their relationship as "wonderful."

She attributed her progress in life to her mother, "who managed to convey that I was well loved whether she was around or not." As to her sister, she felt they "got along fine" except that she found her dull and boring. On the whole, Lillian had made peace with her family.

Regarding Chestnut Lodge, Lillian emphasized that hospitalization was her choice and said "institutions are easy for me . . . the structure made more sense than the structure at home." She felt that if she could have gone to a boarding school during high school, she might have had fewer problems, citing her good adjustments at summer camp in childhood as an example.

She explained that she was dysfunctional prior to the hospitalization and unable to perform "everyday things" and that she needed to be in a place to "rearrange my thought processes." Lillian also felt she had suffered from a postpartum depression, as had both her mother and grandmother.

She expressed fragments of ideas as to other difficulties that led to the hospital: her parents were hypocrites and their values didn't coincide with hers; she always had enormous amounts of energy that she wasn't able to channel effectively; she was a "truth seer," which drove others crazy and got her into trouble; "a child wasn't supposed to know those things."

Lillian was emphatic about what helped her: her high motivation, Dr. Peters, and the structure he provided. Unlike all her previous therapists, Dr. Peters had a "strong enough personality." She recalled him saying to her, "I'm not paid to care about you, I'm paid to treat you." This, she felt, was what she needed to hear. This kept her from "veering too far." In contrast, she felt that her first therapist, Dr. Richards, "let me get away with anything and was a marshmallow." She saw the months with Dr. Davis as a "holding action" and continued to speak with some contempt that he had let himself be drafted. She expressed her beliefs about choosing doctors quite vehemently and concluded that "unless one has a doctor one feels good about, therapy is useless."

Lillian had no idea how Dr. Peters felt toward her, although she speculated that he was relatively "pleased that the analysis was more successful than not." Lillian summed the process of psychotherapy as "dredging out all of the things that didn't make sense . . . like . . . putting together a jigsaw puzzle of your whole life and when the pieces don't fit you shove them in wrong and they are real hard to get out and you have to take the whole thing apart and start all over . . . sorting it all out for myself to determine my own views."

She confirmed that there were other hospital experiences that helped. She recalled her relationship with Robert as highly therapeutic. For the first time she was able to observe herself in a relationship and discuss it. Lillian also believed that she excelled in hospital activities that she had been unable to do at school. These successes gave her confidence in her abilities and strengthened her self-esteem. In retrospect, Lillian felt that Chestnut Lodge had helped her to find "somewhere inside myself that I could be peaceful with anything that came up in my life." She had developed a core sense of self-esteem, comfort, and confidence within herself.

DISCUSSION OF ETIOLOGY AND OUTCOME OF DISORDER

Lillian had one of the best outcomes of the Chestnut Lodge BPD pa-tients studied, and her level of disorder was the mildest. We hypothe-size that her good outcome was related to having the fewest risk factors and the best protective factors, as elaborated below.

Etiology

Biological and Environmental Risk Factors

The biological risk factors that contributed to the development of the disorder included a family history of depression, anxiety, eating disor-ders, and alcoholism. Cluster B traits were apparent in the "holy terror" grandmother and the highly successful and charismatic grandfather and in both parents. Father appeared to have a significant personality disturbance that interfered with work and interpersonal relationships. Mother had considerable narcissistic vulnerability.

Lillian's temperament at birth was described as difficult, and her early affective and behavioral dysregulation exhibited through "willful" be-haviors indicates the presence of these biological factors and a disor-ganized attachment mode. Under the stress of her mother's absence during illness, Lillian's behavioral strategies collapsed. She also had a reading disability, which, as evidence for an underlying processing problem, contributed to her dissociation and increased frustration at school. The processing problem also contributed to problems with lan-guage development.

Mrs. Rand's frequent illness, Mr. Rand's tuberculosis, and sister Kathy's illness, which further occupied mother's time, all occurred during the first 5 years of Lillian's life. The frequent disruptions and separations in the family resulted in biparental emotional neglect of Lillian's needs during these early years. This included a lack of consistent structure and discipline and a lack of protection. These factors also contributed to the inadequate development of a "good enough" goal-corrected partnership that would have helped Lillian develop an emotional vocabulary and emotional and behavioral regulation. Also, during latency and adolescence, Mr. Rand was unable to maintain an appropriate parental role. His behaviors were more those of a competitive sibling or petty tyrant, contributing to ongoing emotional abuse.

The troubled marital relationship of Lillian's parents served as a chronic stressor. They exhibited similarities in personality and temperament in that they were extraverted, social, and highly expressive while sharing underlying feelings of inadequacy and helplessness. However, their adaptive styles were contradictory; father alternated between screaming anger or passive defeat and was a work failure, although with a facade of respectability; mother was well organized and highly competent socially, although overburdened by full responsibility for the family. They could not support each other and provide united parental guidance and structure, a sufficient holding environment, for Lillian's developmental needs. Father was in a sense the more typically feminine partner despite his sportsmanship, letting Mrs. Rand run the family. Their opposite styles must have confused and overwhelmed Lillian and made it difficult to develop a cohesive identity. Although Lillian adopted what appears to be a masculine identity, she may actually have identified with her more competent mother.

Protective Factors

There were many protective factors with Lillian's case and with her family that were ameliorative. Despite her reading disability, Lillian had high intelligence. She was engaging and lively and had an infectious sense of humor. She also had considerable artistic talent. Further, her experiences during latency while at summer camp enabled her to develop the experience of success as a result of concentrated effort. Her camp experience also helped her to develop her peer abilities and overall sense of competence. Although Lillian led a double life in high school, her ability to interact with and get along with a wide range of peers and to enjoy success in extracurricular activities further helped her to develop her abilities. These experiences later contributed to her substantial professional success.

The Rands were neither malicious nor mean. Mrs. Rand overall was a "good enough" mother, as evidenced by her determined attempt to nurse Lillian and do the right thing developmentally. She persevered in her attempts to organize resources for her family and provide for the special needs of both daughters. Lillian verified this during the follow-up interview when she stated that she always knew her mother loved and supported her. Thus, the biparental neglect present during parts of Lillian's childhood was not persistent and was related primarily to family illness and her father's personality disturbance and alcoholism. Her mother's ability to hire good live-in help to assist in the caregiving of the children made a real difference. Minna was apparently a reliable and sensitive caregiver to whom Lillian felt close and who was able to reduce the disruption within the family.

Both parents sought professional help for themselves, and her mother made repeated attempts to obtain professional help for Lillian. Mother's social and organizational competence was a good model for Lillian. The family had a wide network of friends and acquaintances in the community. Lillian had extensive support from this network and also additional models for successful living. She was able to generate a similar wide network as an adult.

Outcome

At the time of discharge, Lillian was greatly improved and able to function in the world and continue her development as a young adult. The hospital provided her with the kind of consistent, reliable structure and support that a good home does. Within this environment Lillian's natural abilities and capacities could flourish. She took advantage of the occupational and art therapies available to further solidify her creative abilities that later led to much success in the world.

Cognitive Dysfunction

Lillian's cognitive processing problems, as indicated by her reading disability, probably contributed to the degree of dissociation she exhibited. Dissociation appeared early and was prevalent throughout the course of treatment. At follow-up, Lillian continued to manifest a dissociative quality, as she stated she rarely felt sad or cried. She continued to speak in blunt and simple sentences. Despite her intellectual capacity, she was surprisingly not psychologically minded. Her interest in astrology during the follow-up period supports this. She evidenced minimal understanding of the origins of her problems. It is notable, however, that

Lillian felt that she needed the hospital to "rearrange my thought processes." Thus, she was aware of some form of cognitive reorganization.

Emotional Regulation

Affective instability.   Lillian did suffer from affective instability and was highly reactive to family stress and separation. Lillian also had depression and anxiety that in childhood were expressed through withdrawal and that later appeared postpartum. Although at follow-up she did not report problems with depression or anxiety, we assumed she continued to experience some difficulty, as seen through continued milder problems with substance abuse, eating, and promiscuity. Over the course of the follow-up period, her high energy and her action-oriented style were more effectively directed toward intensive involvement in work and hobbies. Her emotional life, however, seemed somewhat shallow in that she avoided deep emotions related to intimate involvement with others. Her predominant narcissistic style was more effectively organized to regulate affect.

Anger.   Lillian displayed intense anger with frequent displays of temper tantrums from an early age. At follow-up, Lillian described episodic "raging periods," which she treated with overeating or drinking, but commented that these periods had lessened in frequency and intensity. One example of her improved anger management was her ability to "let go" of quarrels with her husband. Her intense anger appeared to have been transformed into a more modulated but nonetheless still abrasive and combative style.

Behavioral Regulation

Impulsive and compulsive use of pleasurable behaviors.   Lillian exhibited the full range of impulsive and compulsive behaviors, including substance abuse, binge eating, and sexual promiscuity, and frantic efforts to avoid abandonment. However, she did not exhibit the recurrent suicidal behavior and self-mutilating characteristics of many patients with BPD. At follow-up, her behavioral regulation demonstrated gradual improvement. During the first half of the follow-up period, Lillian continued to engage in casual sexual liaisons through maintaining an "open" marriage. By the second half, she reported that work had replaced sexual involvements. Lillian continued to have episodic substance abuse problems at follow-up, but she appeared to have gradually brought the substance abuse under better control. She also appeared to have brought her eating disorder under better management, as she indicated her weight swung only 5 instead of 30 pounds.

Unstable Intense Relationships

Lillian exhibited intense, unstable relatedness with her parents, her boy-friends, and her Chestnut Lodge therapist characteristic of a mildy dis-organized attachment mode with preoccupied and dismissing features. Lillian's relationships gradually stabilized over the course of the fol-low-up period related to greater integration and organization of a pre-dominately dismissing-detached attachment mode, although there were many echoes of the young Lillian. Her improvement was maintained and strengthened because of her ability to find an adaptive work and social niche and to find a man with whom she could have a detached mode of attachment. Once they settled on a more distant closeness and she became more involved in work and projects, her emotional and behavioral dysregulation seemed under better control. She maintained a distant closeness with others manifested by her confident, cocky style that eschewed too much emotionality.

Identity Diffusion

At home and at Chestnut Lodge, Lillian had developed a social identity as a deviant truthsayer who exposed pretension and sham, and later she forged a career identity as an executive. Lillian also had a stable het-erosexual identity. Her gender identity, however, was more mixed. Lil-lian viewed herself as the predator in sexual relationships, and her promiscuity suggested more typically masculine than feminine identi-fication, as did her rejection of motherhood. This identity further stabi-lized along these lines over the follow-up period. Her masculine gender identification solidified with a career as a successful and brash execu-tive, nonchalant sexual liaisons, and adamant rejection of motherhood. The dismissing attachment mode—that is, maintaining attachment through minimizing the importance of attachment—is also more typi-cal of male borderline patients in the Chestnut Lodge BPD sample. This predominant identity resulted in acceptance into the corporate culture, where assertiveness and decisiveness are virtues. Lillian's feminine identity was, nonetheless, evident in her choice of the fashion industry and her interest in home design and crafts.

DISCUSSION OF TREATMENT

We elaborate more fully on the universal features and recurrent issues and themes in treatment as illustrated by the cases in Chapters 7 ("Uni-versal Features of Treatment") and 8 ("Recurrent Themes and Issues").

However, after each case history, we highlight briefly the following aspects of the treatment: 1) comparison with current-day treatments, 2) therapeutic factors, 3) countertherapeutic factors, and 4) therapist struggles.

Comparison With Current Treatments

The most glaring omission in Lillian's treatment, by today's standards, was the use of antidepressants for her postpartum depression. However, those medications were not available at the time. If Lillian could have been treated immediately with antidepressants, it might have prevented or slowed her dramatic downward spiral. Also, a brief hospitalization or crisis residential stay along with medications might have been sufficient to stabilize her so that she could, once again, use outpatient psychotherapy. Involvement in some form of concurrent substance abuse treatment would also be recommended. Another important part of the treatment plan would include assessment of her reading disability and a remediation plan. Finally, a structured family therapy, both before entry into Chestnut Lodge and during her stay, might have been very helpful. Lillian's first therapist was very supportive of the family, accepting crisis phone calls and giving advice, but did not attempt family therapy.

Today, there would be standard inquiry into the presence of sexual abuse in Lillian's history both during the initial evaluation and during the course of therapy. Lillian expressed concerns about rape and described how she trembled at her father's touch. With our increased understanding of the role of child abuse in the development of the disorder, these concerns would have been explored in a different way.

Therapeutic Factors

Although the additional treatment interventions outlined above would have been helpful and perhaps sufficient, we feel they would not have addressed Lillian's need for ongoing structure and containment. She needed the village and asylum provided at Chestnut Lodge, or as she stated, the boarding school and summer camp structure. Her home had been too chaotic to provide such structure. The containment and "holding" provided at Chestnut Lodge enabled her to regulate her emotions and behaviors for a sufficiently long time period that she could fully engage in therapy and the opportunities available at Chestnut Lodge. She was able to "excel" in art and occupational activities and for the first time experience success. This helped her to build her self-esteem and confidence and to develop knowledge and skills she could later apply to daily living and in a work setting.

Because three different psychiatrists treated Lillian, we can see the cumulative effects of treatment and how therapeutic experiences can build on one another. Of major importance was the therapeutic alliance. As Lillian said, "Unless one has a doctor one feels good about, therapy is useless." Dr. Richards, her first therapist, by his own report provided a very active and supportive approach with "strong confrontation and direct interpretation." With his help, Lillian was able to graduate from high school and maintain the forward course of development. His active, "here and now" stance served to stabilize her through adolescence and to minimize the disruption to regular development. However, she had not internalized their relationship enough to sustain her when she left home to attend school. Without therapeutic assistance, she quickly deteriorated into promiscuity and alcohol abuse. This parallels the course of BPD in many patients in that they can maintain functioning while in treatment but once the structure and support (i.e., a stable attachment) are gone they often are unable to regulate emotion and behavior under stressful conditions.

Both Dr. Davis and Dr. Peters enjoyed Lillian's sense of humor. She was "extremely, infectiously amusing" and could dilute a tense moment with a wry comment. Dr. Peters attributed his ability to persevere to Lillian's sense of humor. The use of humor, when present in therapist and patient, is an important feature in maintaining the alliance.

Lillian's description of her first psychiatrist at Chestnut Lodge, Dr. Davis, as the "marshmallow" highlights the BPD patient's need to perceive their therapist as competent and sturdy. We suspect that her view of him was colored by his being drafted and leaving her. He was quickly devalued, perhaps as her way to protect herself from the loss. However, she did not appear to have a "good enough" working alliance with him, as she emphasized that "he let me get away with anything," underscoring the need for clear limits and containment.

Dr. Peters, the "strong enough" therapist, was what she needed. She valued his no-nonsense, "I'm not paid to care about you but paid to treat you" stance. Of course, he did like and care for her, which made a difference. But his ability to keep her from "veering too far" was the necessary condition for good treatment. Her description of therapy as "putting together a jigsaw puzzle of your whole life and when the pieces don't fit you shove them in wrong . . . you have to take the whole thing apart and start all over" captures the therapeutic work of integration. All of her therapists established a relationship characterized by a goal-corrected partnership in which they engaged in a dialogue about thoughts, feelings, longings, and wishes that enabled her to construct a shared world and a personal narrative.

Another important feature of the treatment was Dr. Peters's willingness to see her for extra sessions and accept phone calls during times of increased need and suicidal feelings. This was illustrated by his behavior following the anniversary of her child's adoption and the loss of her boyfriend.

Further, she noted that being able to discuss her romantic relationship with a fellow patient in therapy was extremely useful. We suspect that here, too, the fact that the relationship was conducted within Chestnut Lodge and monitored by staff, similar to the way a parent monitors an adolescent's relationships, made a difference. The stability of the attachment with her therapist reduced the intensity of her need in a dependent relationship and enabled her to better observe herself.

Countertherapeutic Factors

Two sequences in treatment illustrate possible countertherapeutic activity. When Dr. Peters, worn down by Lillian's "childish, whiny, and demanding" requests to leave the hospital, confronted her whining, she became quite disorganized. We wondered if what disorganized her may have been Dr. Peters's underlying anger and impatience in tone rather than his actual words. When BPD patients perceive criticism/judgment and feel pushed away in a significant relationship, they can become disorganized. Lillian's whining behavior was an expression of both her intense dependence on Dr. Peters and feelings of helplessness and anger over his having so much perceived control. A confrontation of behavior rather than discussion of what motivated it is a common mistake in therapy with BPD patients. Also, Lillian's persistent whining and nagging may have indicated a disruption in the relationship. She was reenacting the behavior she engaged in to get attention from her father. Dr. Peters may have neglected to attend to some aspects of Lillian's emotional needs of which both were unaware.

Another possible countertherapeutic response was Dr. Peters's silence in response to her requests to know more about him. This is a fundamental question for BPD patients. The therapist is often experienced as depersonalized and unknowable because the patient has never known herself or her parents in an integrated fashion. The therapist is really being asked, "Who are you in relation to me?" What kind of a person are you . . . trustworthy?" and "How does this business of being in a relationship work?" Also, silence is rarely a helpful response to BPD patients and often disorganizes them. They jump too quickly to a paranoid or abusive interpretation of silence.

Therapist Struggles

Although Dr. Richards, Lillian's psychiatrist during high school, did not reveal his personal feelings toward Lillian, we gleaned from his summary that he cared for and understood her. However, once she returned home from college, he clearly began feeling out of control and frightened for her safety. It was perhaps Dr. Richards's loss of confidence in his ability to treat her combined with the parents' panic that pushed the hospitalization. Also, Lillian's family was quite prominent in the community, and he had a close relationship with them. He undoubtedly was unwilling to risk Lillian's further destructive behavior out of concern for both Lillian and his reputation. The heightened risk that BPD patients pose to therapists and psychiatrists can sometime interfere with adequate treatment or lead them to terminate their treatment prematurely.

At the Chestnut Lodge case conference, staff expressed concern over "boundaries," expressed primarily as how much involvement there should be with Lillian's family. Also, both Chestnut Lodge psychiatrists periodically felt sexually seduced by Lillian. Although neither appeared unduly concerned with this aspect of Lillian's behavior, a concern with boundaries is common in work with BPD patients. BPD patients are at high risk for sexual misconduct by therapists, and therapists are at high risk for false accusations of sexual misconduct by BPD patients. Therapists are more likely to violate professional ethics with BPD patients than with patients in any other diagnostic group, as will be discussed further in Chapter 8.

Dr. Peters often questioned himself and his effectiveness. So convincing were Lillian's devaluing attacks that he felt increasingly inadequate. This feeling of inadequacy is a frequent response to the BPD patient and underscores the importance of collegial support and consultation.

4

Love Having No Geography...Susan

The brain may take advice but not the heart
and love having no geography
knows no boundaries

Truman Capote, Other Voices, Other Rooms

On her eighteenth birthday, Susan, a tall, blond, striking young woman fled from her first hospital treatment against medical advice (AMA). She desperately sought reunion with her boyfriend but, on being rejected by him, threw herself into a river hoping to die. Rescued by the police, she was hospitalized at Chestnut Lodge, where she remained for the next 3 years.

HISTORY OF DISORDER

The first time overt problems were observed was when Susan entered kindergarten. Teachers identified a "nervous problem," and her pediatrician prescribed phenobarbital. Susan's problems next became apparent in the fourth grade at the time of her mother's first serious suicide attempt. Susan was described at the time as shy, tense, anxious, and often sucking her fingers. The school recommended psychological testing, but this was never pursued. When Susan was 11 and a sixth grader, she discovered her mother unconscious from a drug overdose. At Susan's urging, her father hospitalized her mother. Susan subsequently failed at school and was asked to leave.

In response to her mother's hospitalization and Susan's school failure, her father decided to forge a new life apart from his wife's wealthy family. He took Susan and her sister, Ann, from his in-law's extensive estate to an apartment and found a teaching position in a local high school. Susan transferred to his school in the seventh grade. Although she started in the "bright" group, Susan was quickly demoted to the "stupid" group. This was particularly upsetting, as her father was a much-admired teacher there. She had few, if any, friends and felt quite isolated.

To bolster her father's dream of a new life, one independent of wealthy in-laws and the demoralizing impact of his affair with his sister-in-law, Susan was forced to assume a maternal role. She attempted to keep house and care for her younger sister. This overburdened her slim resources, and she became increasingly numb and depersonalized. Like Lillian (see Chapter 3), she discovered that sexual involvement brought her out of a dissociative state and made her feel more in contact. From this point on, she engaged almost continuously in sexual relationships. She also began relying heavily on alcohol and drugs, especially when disappointed by boyfriends.

In the tenth grade, Susan experienced a brief respite from this pattern. Her grades improved, and she went out for the track team and enjoyed some girlfriends. She developed a close relationship with her coach and won a medal in the state track championship. Later, in her therapy at Chestnut Lodge, she talked fondly of her coach and followed the course of her old team. This was one of the few memories she had of a normal childhood.

This brief period ended abruptly when her mother was discharged from the hospital and asked that her family move near her so she could continue aftercare with the same psychiatrist. Susan became depressed and withdrawn and entered treatment for the first time.

As her behavior became increasingly out of control and self-destructive, Susan's parents fought bitterly over discipline. Her father imposed strict limits, whereas her mother was lenient. Susan spiraled further into drunkenness and promiscuity. Unable to exert any control over her behavior and barely maintaining their own stability, the parents hospitalized Susan.

At this hospital, Susan was described as "passive, pliant, submissive, withdrawn and unreflective." Her doctor felt that she was biding her time until her eighteenth birthday, when she could sign herself out. Immediately following her birthday, however, Susan became drunk and assaultive and had to be placed in restraints and put in seclusion.

Subsequent to this she eloped with another patient but returned under parental pressure. A legal hold was considered but decided against, and Susan left the hospital. Two weeks later she threw herself into a river and was admitted to Chestnut Lodge.

FAMILY HISTORY

Susan's maternal great-grandfather was an inventor, industrialist, and market manipulator who built a fortune that supported subsequent generations. His daughter Carmen, Susan's grandmother, was described as a "beautiful, unstable woman with an omnivorous sexual appetite." She had three marriages and innumerable affairs. When living alone, she suffered bouts of depression and sought psychiatric treatment.

Susan's mother, Grace, never knew her father, who left when she was 3 years of age. She received little care from her two stepfathers. Grace's life as a child was ruled by the endless drama of Carmen's escapades. After Grace gave birth to Susan, she developed a postpartum depression and medicated herself with amphetamines and alcohol, twin addictions that plagued her throughout life. Grace attempted suicide twice when Susan was growing up, the second attempt resulting in a 3-year hospitalization. She remained in some form of psychotherapy and took medications the rest of her life. Staff at Chestnut Lodge described Grace as looking and acting like a schoolgirl. It was difficult to distinguish, when she and Susan were together, who was mother and who daughter.

Susan's father, Steven, was the fifth and only son of six children, from a poor immigrant Irish family. Steven's father was an ironworker who drank heavily and deserted the family. Steven, his mother's favorite child, became the star of his high school track team and president of his class. He attended college on a track scholarship. Throughout Susan's childhood he alternated between living off the great-grandfather's money and working as a tradesman or teacher. Steven also engaged in a long-term affair with Susan's aunt Cynthia, her mother's sister, which continuously destabilized the marriage and family life. He also had a fierce temper, and during one fight attempted to strangle his wife. These outbursts diminished over time and were replaced by depressive episodes. Although involved sporadically in psychotherapy and briefly in psychoanalysis, he committed suicide at the age of 52, three years after Susan left Chestnut Lodge.

Susan's parents met while Steven was in college and Grace was working in her first and only job. The maternal grandparents were bitterly opposed to the marriage because of the difference in social background, but after the marriage they built a home for the newlyweds on the family estate.

DEVELOPMENTAL HISTORY

Susan was born 2 years after her parents married. The pregnancy was normal, and the delivery was uncomplicated. Susan was reported to be a beautiful baby and favored by Carmen, also a beauty. She was also described as a perfect baby who never cried at night and who would lie in bed quietly until her parents awakened. A submissive toddler, Susan did everything she was asked.

When Susan was 21 months old, her sister, Ann, was born. Ann was immediately described as "ugly" by grandmother Carmen, who recommended plastic surgery. Grace, who felt like the ugly duckling in comparison to her beautiful mother, became protective. From this point on, Susan became her father and grandmother's favorite, while Ann was her mother's. Ann was described as quite opposite to Susan: willful, stubborn, and argumentative. Ann and her mother engaged in frequent struggles. Susan, feeling neglected, turned increasingly toward her father.

At the age 3, Susan developed unusual behavior. She would suddenly and unexpectedly begin to race around the house excitedly doing gymnastic-like tricks. This was referred to in the record as "sudden hyperactivity."

Susan's academic work was poor from the beginning. She was considered "dumb," and her educator father berated her frequently for being "stupid." During Susan's early childhood the family lived on a huge estate in the country. Isolated from the community, Susan had as playmates only her sister and the children of the estate caretakers. Despite this, Susan's beauty and pleasant demeanor enabled her to get along relatively well with school peers.

COURSE IN TREATMENT AT CHESTNUT LODGE

When Susan's psychotherapist, Dr. Knowles, first met her, Susan was frightened and reserved. Her face was covered with scratches and bruises from her suicide attempt. He described her as someone who could be attractive "if she would only smile." Her characteristic expression was impassive and bovine, which was in contrast to the drama of her recent suicide attempt. Dr. Knowles initially identified her major difficulty as an inability to express affect. He saw this inhibition leading to bursts of expression in the therapeutic hour and to impulsive behavior outside of the hour.

During her first months at Chestnut Lodge, Susan alternated between being a good, quiet, and withdrawn patient and being rebellious and out of control. When upset, she would jump on the tables and run around the ward in a fashion reminiscent of her hyperactive periods as a preschooler. To the unit staff this also represented ignorance of social conventions or the "poor manners" of an undisciplined rich girl. Staff noted that the more anxious or depressed she became, the more she giggled and the less sense she made. Strong emotions appeared to overwhelm her fragile cognitive structure and resulted in disorganization.

Within 2 months of admission, Susan became involved with a male patient, Joe. Dr. Knowles described the relationship as sadomasochistic in that Susan was slavishly devoted to Joe, whereas he was cavalier and dismissive toward her. Their public kissing, against hospital rules, resulted in her loss of privileges and confinement to the ward.

During her therapy hours, Susan railed against these restrictions. She called nursing staff "cruel and heartless" and tried to enlist milieu aides to circumvent the rules. She felt all of her problems would be solved if she could leave and live with Joe. During this period she "manipulated everyone," was "rebellious and complaining," and presented herself as a victim. Dr. Knowles confronted her focus on establishing who was right and wrong as keeping her from concentrating on her own contributions to these conflicts. This "confused" her. She was unable to specify any personal responsibility beyond reiterating that she had trouble getting along with others. Dr. Knowles then filled in the blanks and enumerated the ways she initiated tensions, until she broke down sobbing, asking him to stop.

Following this session, Susan became more open in her expressions of anger toward Dr. Knowles, experiencing him alternately as a harsh and punitive father and as a negligent mother. At the same time she became increasingly depressed and self-deprecatory. She spent whole sessions talking about how "dumb, ugly, vague, moldable, stupid, compliant, inadequate in conversation, indecisive and fearful" she was— that is, the "all bad" view of herself.

In the seventh month of treatment, Susan began expressing positive feelings toward Dr. Knowles. She told him that his absence for a few days depressed her and left her feeling as though no one cared. This open expression of attachment and dependence extended to the unit, where Susan was now seen as "clinging." She developed such special relationships with two of the ward staff that her fellow patients exhorted her to find age-appropriate peers. Although feeling criticized by their comments, Susan appreciated their concern and no longer reacted with rage.

Susan began a sexual relationship with Joe, although this was against hospital rules. Susan confessed this to Dr. Knowles, which resulted in her restriction to the ward. She became more withdrawn and depressed and sullenly expressed anger toward Dr. Knowles.

Dr. Edwards, who was Susan's administrative doctor and managed the milieu aspects of her care, focused on "dealing with her passivity and extreme constriction of affect" that left her vulnerable to outbursts of rage and self-destructive behavioral enactments. All her emotions would combine, compound each other, and erupt. He also noted that Susan could not negotiate with staff for privileges or activities, suggesting an inability to identify, articulate, and advocate her needs. Dr. Edwards's position was that as much time as was necessary would be allotted to give Susan "the opportunity to gradually unfold." To engineer this, the ward staff kept her restricted and waited for her to initiate any changes. They responded to her "timorous advances with cautious support." Staff remained available to hear her expressions of anger, resentment, and disapproval and to discuss and validate them as needed. Within this milieu, Susan gradually articulated her discontents without enacting them. As this occurred, she began to find more energy for other activities. She became less "vacant and more alert . . . less constricted and manifested an increasing capacity to tolerate depressive affects." She expressed a desire to work and involved herself at the hospital store. She began to state her angry feelings more directly to Dr. Knowles. However, this often left her feeling morose, defeated, and hopeless. After 14 months of treatment, much of it spent restricted to the ward, Susan described feelings of fearfulness and anxiety when allowed unescorted privileges to her therapy hour. She felt alone and insecure. At these times she thought about going "against the rules," feeling secure that she would be "caught" and taken back into restricted status. Susan looked forward to the idea of being watched and cared for more closely. She held the hospital record for length of time on restriction.

Susan also had thoughts of running away whenever Dr. Knowles noted how well she was doing and how therapy was helping her. She feared that being positive about the therapy and her progress meant she no longer needed help and would be thrown from the nest prematurely. Despite these anxieties, Susan gradually became "more autonomous" and began spending nights in an apartment owned by her parents. She eventually increased her time out to the full 7 nights per week. She moved to outpatient status and also began clerking at a local store.

In psychotherapy Susan began to exhibit an ability to elaborate on her thoughts and feelings about Dr. Knowles. In one session, she mentioned that she had not seen Dr. Knowles's car in the parking lot. With great embarrassment, she said, "I hoped you hadn't given it away. I'd love to have it for myself." Another session was preceded by Dr. Knowles opening the door to find Susan lighting a male friend's cigarette. After much silence and hesitation in the hour, she said, "You will think I'm crazy over what I'm going to say. It is a bad thing to think. I wanted you to be jealous. Isn't that awful?" This confession led to a tirade of self-denigration. Nevertheless, it was a clear sign of her increased ability to recognize and express feelings within the psychotherapeutic context.

Trouble, however, was not far away. Two weeks after her transition to outpatient status, Dr. Knowles learned that Susan was dating a former hospital aide, Grant. One of the staff had seen them together. This also was against hospital rules. Dr. Knowles informed Susan of this, and after a long silence she confessed to the relationship and asked Dr. Knowles what he thought. He was silent. Susan wondered aloud why she had been so secretive and said, "It must be from the past." She expressed a desire to avoid keeping secrets and said the relationship was important to her and different from any relationship in her past. Dr. Knowles remained silent for the remainder of the session, as did Susan. The next two sessions were also largely silent. Toward the end of these, Susan expressed concern that treatment could not go on.

Susan's staff case conference was held at this time. The medical staff was divided over the meaning of Susan's behavior and how to respond. Some staff members felt that her relationship with Grant was a means of maintaining the tie with the hospital as she separated. Others were concerned that her behavior was a cry for a return to inpatient status. Dr. Knowles was advised to abandon his silence, which Susan might interpret as disinterest and neglect. He was further urged to present a "real person aspect" and to express a strong reaction to her behavior and bring her back into the hospital.

Dr. Knowles followed this advice and readmitted her to the hospital. At first, Susan seemed "obviously reassured," but 1 month later she went AWOL. She resumed her relationship with Grant but maintained contact with the hospital by telephone. Within 3 weeks, Susan returned to the hospital, and over the next month she terminated contact with Grant, obtained a secretarial position at the hospital, and regained full privileges. She found work as a bus girl at a Holiday Inn and was promoted to waitress. She planned to renew her driver's test and buy a car for work.

In the context of these developments, Susan resumed her relationship with Grant. She was secretive about it at first. Soon, however, she became openly angry with staff and with Dr. Knowles. She decided to leave the hospital within 3 days. A discharge AMA was arranged, and therapy was discontinued.

FOLLOW-UP SEVEN YEARS LATER

At follow-up 7 years later, Susan was 28 years old and living alone in her own apartment. She was in the process of moving back to her hometown to be near her mother and a man she had recently begun dating. She agreed to an extended in-person interview and was seen on two separate occasions.

The interviewer described her as stunning woman who could have been a model. The interviewer's first impression was of a "dumb blonde," as her responses were simple, often imprecise, and ingenuous. As the interview progressed, this impression was dispelled. She communicated in a sincere, thoughtful, and frequently insightful manner.

Aftercare Treatment

A year after discharge from Chestnut Lodge, Susan restarted her therapy with Dr. Knowles because, as she said, "I was having a rough time." She saw him as a private patient four to five times weekly over the next 5 years. While in treatment, she had one psychiatric hospitalization about a year later. This hospitalization followed a breakup of a relationship and her father's suicide. Unemployed, she spent her days at her apartment drinking to oblivion. Dr. Knowles prescribed Elavil to treat her depression, but she was unable to stop her alcohol use. One day she took too much of both and overdosed. She awakened in the early morning and, realizing what she had done, called Dr. Knowles. He hospitalized her for 3 weeks at a community hospital.

Relationships

Six months after her AMA discharge, Susan married Grant. She said, in retrospect, "I loved him . . .[,] needed him (and) depended greatly on him." She reconstructed her departure from Chestnut Lodge as a scary and lonely time and said, "Everyone was against me, and I thought I was all alone in this world." Because of this, she "latched" onto Grant. They were married for 2½ stormy years. She found herself intensely jealous and would lash out at him physically when drunk. Both engaged in extramarital affairs. Eventually Susan left the relationship, stating she could not stand the fighting and the feeling that their "ideas on life" were so different.

Immediately after their separation, Susan became involved with Grant's best and married friend, Alvin, for whom Susan had been working. This prompted Alvin's separation from his wife and many hard feelings among the four former friends. Susan and Alvin remained sexually involved for 2 years. After Alvin, she dated a variety of men, one of whom she referred to as a "very nice man," another as the "one I went to Mexico with . . . he was Fall to Spring."

At follow-up, Susan noted she had more male than female friends. Most of these relationships were sexual. Her most recent relationship was with the mayor of the small town where her mother lived. Although they had only known each other for 2 months, she was willing to move there to be closer. She felt it was different from her other relationships. She experienced greater "rapport and give and take." He was someone to marry and with whom to have children. Nevertheless, although she planned to move and develop this relationship, she maintained casual sexual relationships with her other male friends.

Socially, most of Susan's time was spent with her male friends. She eschewed female friendships to avoid "the intensity." Perhaps her closest companions were two cats, whom she referred to as "my joys in life." She recalled with sorrow having taken two cats to the pound during the first year of her marriage. Forced to move into a building that did not permit pets, she had no alternative. She spent many therapy hours lamenting her action and still felt guilty.

Work

After discharge Susan continued as a waitress for a few months and over the next several years held a series of "little jobs" interspersed with secretarial work for Alvin. These jobs were part-time, and none lasted longer than nine months. Later, she obtained a job as a secretary. Her hours were variable and depended on her emotional state, but she worked regularly for 4 years. Overall, she felt pleased with her performances. Her family's money supported her throughout, but Susan took pride in being able to contribute.

Substance Use

Susan's alcohol use fluctuated over the follow-up period. After discharge, she drank heavily and had one nearly fatal car accident while intoxicated. Drinking also disinhibited her, and she could become physically assaultive. At one point, she stopped drinking and substituted marijuana, which helped her to "remain calm." However, she soon found herself dependent, so she reserved the marijuana for "medicinal" use when she felt "hyper" and could not sleep. In its place she resumed drinking a cocktail in the evening. She considered her current alcohol use recreational. About her prior heavy drinking, she said, "I tried to drown myself, so I couldn't feel myself and my mind."

Mood Lability

Susan noted that her worst episode of "hyperactivity" occurred at Chestnut Lodge and resulted in treatment with sheet packs. She recalled that she would get "crazy high" talking, laughing, and joking. She added, "I would get very depressed for a period of time. . . . I couldn't stand it anymore so I would go the other way. I will take being hyper over being depressed any day."

She reported that her ups and downs continued but were "less intense." She no longer felt suicidal and stated that her suicide attempt left her "terrified" of dying. She said, "After my father's suicide [I realized] there is no point to that. . . . I know I'll get old and my time will come." Susan felt she had learned how to express anger at Chestnut Lodge and how to identify different mood states. In describing her views about hospitalization, Susan said, "I needed to leave home, and that's how I did it." She felt that the experience at Chestnut Lodge provided her with a "foundation." Susan's favorite, "most therapeutic" person at the Lodge, next to Dr. Knowles, was a female aide, Minerva, "a great big African-American woman with eleven children" who had worked at the hospital for many years. Susan's description of their relationship was revealing. She stated:

> Every time Minerva came on duty I would run up and give her a big hug . . . I would talk to her no matter what. I was really depressed[;] we would sit down and play cards . . . we didn't do too much talking . . . she let me be myself. Sometimes I would get really high and act really goofy but she would just handle it . . . she was a mother image . . . my mother was sick for so many years.

Whereas Minerva was like a mother, Susan said Dr. Knowles helped her to "learn about myself." Her feelings toward Dr. Knowles were deep and abiding. Her work with him "made the difference between [mere] existence and a [full] life for me. . . . I feel I can have a meaningful life."

Through her treatment with Dr. Knowles she felt she had developed the ability to think logically. She stated, "[When] my emotions come up and they are too involved . . . I use some power in the brain to push things aside and just think and then I can do whatever the situation (requires) . . . I come out with a strength within myself, and I know I can handle whatever."

DISCUSSION OF ETIOLOGY AND OUTCOME OF DISORDER

Susan's disorder was moderately severe. It corresponds with moderate biological vulnerability in interaction with moderate environmental stressors and some important protective factors.

Etiology

Biological and Environmental Risk Factors

A history of depression, alcoholism, and Cluster B personality disorders existed on both sides of Susan's family. The degree of mental illness in the family is highlighted by father's suicide and mother's continuous hospitalizations. Grandparents and parents exhibited Cluster B traits, and mother and grandmother appeared to fit the general criteria for BPD and histrionic personality disorders. The family's interrelationships were incestuous and chaotic, and there was barely a semblance of an orderly structured home life. Susan's early life was characterized by persistent biparental neglect of her developmental needs. Mother was mostly absent or at best a sister; father tried to keep the family together but was unable to maintain a consistent home life and parentified Susan. Further, he demeaned and devalued Susan's intelligence and school perfor-mance. Susan witnessed her parent's frequent fighting and their inabil-ity to agree over her parenting. As with Lillian (see Chapter 3), there was no opportunity for the parents to develop a goal-corrected partnership with Susan earlier or later in her development. Further, the family's self-absorption and physical distance from the community provided mini-mal opportunity for Susan to develop peer relationships.

Protective Factors

Despite the many failures within this family system, there were strengths and protective factors as well. First, the family lived within a commu-nity in which they were prominent and active and had a positive identity. There was no evidence of bizarre or psychotic-like thinking in either the maternal or paternal sides of the family. Communications were crude but straightforward. Mother seemed to care for her daughters and lacked malice or cruelty. Both parents kept trying to get their lives in or-der: father through work, therapy, and attempts at independence from his wife's family; mother through extensive therapy, both inpatient and day treatment. We imagine that their continuous efforts to improve their lives provided a model for Susan to persevere in her therapy and life, with the tragic exception of her father's ultimate suicide. However, even with this heartrending loss, Susan drew further motivation to improve her life.

Susan's beauty and apparent likeability served as a protective factor. She was able to engage others, particularly men, and maintain their involvement in a relationship. Also, she had developed a modicum of self-discipline and ability to work—perhaps related to the years she spent alone with her father trying to care for the household and her younger sister.

Outcome

Susan's outcome was moderately successful. She appeared to have developed a more organized and stable preoccupied attachment pattern with men and avoided relationships with women, resulting in fewer periods of disorganization and greater behavioral and emotional regulation. Nonetheless, she retained significant developmental immaturity in most areas.

Cognitive Dysfunction

Susan, like Lillian, experienced depersonalized states as a child and into adolescence and young adulthood. Sexual involvement was her method of restoring feeling. Susan's intellectual functioning was normal (Wechsler Adult Intelligence Scale: Verbal IQ = 107; Performance IQ = 99), but she impressed others as dumb. We felt that this misperception was related both to Susan's dissociation and to her inarticulateness. Susan's simple language revealed her rudimentary conceptualizations of self and others. She demonstrated naive psychological constructs about her motivations. As with Lillian, therapists noted that under stress Susan made "no sense," indicating that her elementary cognitive schemas were easily disrupted.

At follow-up, Susan did not describe dissociative states. Instead, she appeared much more able to describe and differentiate emotional states. Even so, Susan still conveyed an impression of inarticulateness. She continued to speak in rudimentary psychological terms, and her use of language was adolescent.

Emotional Regulation

Affective instability.   Susan suffered throughout her life with being either very low or "crazy high." Her early "hyperactivity" and subsequent "nervous" problem point toward an unstable mood but also may have been a manifestation of disorganized attachment. Throughout adolescence she struggled with depression and anxiety. At follow-up, she said her highs and lows were "less intense" but an enduring aspect of her life. She also had been treated with antidepressants.

Intense anger and lack of control of anger. Susan was described as "nervous," docile, and withdrawn throughout most of her childhood. Her anger became apparent during her hospitalizations. She reportedly lost her temper with staff when she was restricted to the unit. Alcohol ignited her anger, as evidenced by physical fights with boyfriends. During the follow-up period, frequent uncontrollable physical and verbal fights marked Susan's first marriage. However, later in the follow-up period, Susan emphasized her dislike of intense anger. There was a gradual decrease in the intensity with which she experienced anger and a newly developed ability to modulate.

Behavioral Regulation

Impulsive/compulsive use of pleasurable behaviors. Like Lillian, Susan discovered that sex provided an antidote to depersonalized states as early as seventh grade. By most standards, Susan would be deemed promiscuous. She continued to engage in casual sexual affairs during her marriage and throughout the follow-up period while maintaining parallel love relationships.

Susan also continued to struggle with abuse of alcohol and marijuana. However, she appeared to acknowledge and accept her vulnerability toward addiction and made concerted efforts to control it.

Suicidal/self-mutilative behaviors. Susan never engaged in self-mutilation. However, she made at least one purposeful and serious suicide attempt and several suicidal gestures. All these occurred when she was under the influence of drugs and alcohol. When sober, she may have had suicidal ideation but did not act on it. Several years after discharge from Chestnut Lodge, Susan made one serious suicide attempt. However, after her own near lethal attempt and her father's successful suicide, Susan reported an unequivocal decision to live.

Behaviors driven by abandonment fears. Susan reported that when she felt separated and isolated she would experience emptiness and then "act out." The driven quality of her involvement with men suggests that she was trying to avoid feelings related to separation and abandonment.

Unstable Intense Relationships

Susan's attachment pattern, as evident in her relationship with her parents, was moderately disorganized and primarily preoccupied. Mother was absent for long periods of time and mostly neglectful when present. When mother was present, Susan was probably frightened by her partly because of her suicidality and frequent intoxication and out-of-control behavior. When engaged, mother parentified Susan and treated her as confidante and pal. Father alternated between devaluing and belittling Susan's intelligence and competence while placing her prematurely in a caretaking role for her sister and their home. Susan seemed to have adequate superficial relationships with schoolmates. With the onset of puberty, Susan turned to sexual relationships as a means to maintain organization and cope with the effects of long years of deprivation and neglect. Her immaturity and overreliance on these relationships for nurturance resulted in promiscuity that can be understood as a result of her disorganized attachment and a form of behavioral dysregulation. We also suspect that her disinterest in friendships with women was related to a dismissal of them as a source of nurturance. As she indicated, "They become too intense," and relationships with them may have disorganized her even more than did relationships with men. This is not surprising, given her motherless childhood and her father's greater availability.

Susan's first therapeutic relationship was described as sadomasochistic and highly eroticized. Her doctor was characterized as "devoted" to her. His written comments at termination were disappointed and punitive in tone as he wrote, "The last easy escape route from hospitalization that I chose to close was her avenue back into the warm, undemanding security of her home." At Chestnut Lodge, Susan was described as "slavishly" devoted to her boyfriend and devaluing of hospital staff, whom she accused of being cruel and heartless. Staff portrayed Susan as rebellious, complaining, and manipulative. Her relationship with the former hospital aide is typical of the tempestuous relationships BPD patients can form in residential settings and how they engage and "split" an entire staff. Her relationship with Dr. Knowles and the treatment team at Chestnut Lodge was characteristically stormy and ended, typically, with a discharge "against medical advice."

After discharge, Susan's marriage to the hospital aide was highly disorganized and marked by mutual infidelity and drunken violent fights. Her marriage ended chaotically in the midst of an affair with her husband's best and married friend. With continued therapy and life experience, Susan's attachment mode appeared to stabilize to a greater degree, as evidenced by improved emotional and behavioral regulation and less overall disorganization. However, by most cultural standards, she would still be considered unstable. It was of note that she did not refer to her boyfriends by name but by season, "Fall or Spring," or by location of relationship (e.g., "He was Mexico"). Relationships with women continued to be avoided, as they mirrored the relationship with her mother too closely and triggered excessive longing and disappointment. Her plan to live closer to her mother suggests on ongoing attempt to restore the relationship and continued preoccupation.

Identity Disturbance

Susan had a stable heterosexual and gender identity. Her most enduring identity was that of a "beautiful woman," and it was not surprising to learn that her primary identity at follow-up continued to be that of a "beautiful woman who could attract many men." It was her major asset in the world, as it had been her grandmother's.

Although of average intelligence, she was unable to achieve in school, and she graduated with a graduate equivalency degree and suffered with a negative identity as "dumb." Except for her brief success on the school track team, Susan did not demonstrate any special talents or interests, nor did she have an opportunity to develop them. Despite her attempts as family caretaker during mother's hospitalizations, she appeared to try to avoid this role in relationships. However, her experience as caretaker with her father, mother, and younger sister, combined with the structure provided at Chestnut Lodge, may have enabled her to develop a modicum of self-discipline and an ability to work at least part time. Also, she had the example of her father, who continuously attempted to work. At follow-up, she appeared to be pursuing a more traditional course for women of her background, as she accepted support from family money and pursued a possible second marriage.

DISCUSSION OF TREATMENT

Comparison With Current Treatments

Like Lillian, Susan could have benefited from psychopharmacological treatment. Although depressive symptoms predominated, there was also evidence of episodic manic symptoms that at one point were severe enough to warrant sheet packs. She, today, would be involved in some form of substance abuse treatment. Family treatment, focusing on helping the parents learn how to parent and set appropriate limits and discipline, would have been helpful earlier in Susan's life. However, the severity of her mother's disorders and the degree of dysfunction in the marriage would have been a challenge to the best family therapist.

Therapeutic Factors

For Susan, both the residential milieu and the opportunity for long-term psychotherapy seemed important. Susan desperately needed a stable home, a foundation. The hospital milieu could not replace what had never been, but it could work to moderate the negative consequences of her prolonged childhood deprivation. One of the most effective aspects of her care was the treatment team's persistence. That she was on restriction longer than any other patient attests to Susan's need for the experience of being cared for and protected. She needed consistent support and guidance.

Another therapeutic feature that Susan highlighted at follow-up was the opportunity to "be myself." The milieu, in the person of earth mother Minerva, accepted Susan for how she was. Instead of reacting negatively to Susan's depressed or "goofy" behavior, Minerva appeared to respond to the need underneath. She could either be a comforting presence or distract Susan from her sadness by playing cards and thus helping her to learn that a shared activity with a loved one is a good antidote. Minerva also was an important member of the treatment team, and she embodied the mothering qualities that Susan had so sorely missed.

Dr. Knowles engaged Susan in cognitive development through dialogue. This "dumb" young woman developed the ability to think logically. The therapeutic relationship was as important as the milieu. Dr. Knowles exhibited all of the qualities of a good therapist: nonjudgmental, respectful, accepting, patient, genuine, and empathic. This enabled Susan to maintain the relationship and use it as her anchor for further development.

Countertherapeutic Factors

The most negative feature of the treatment was the staff's response to Susan's involvement with Grant, the hospital aide. Although understandable, their response was an overreaction, as was the plan to place a legal hold on her. She was not psychotic, gravely disabled, suicidal, or underage. The threat of a hold was too arbitrary and punitive a response. The team's fierce disapproval, experienced as abandonment, increased Susan's dependence on Grant. Such relationships must run their course and be discussed within therapy.

Therapist Struggles

This same incident was also the major struggle for Dr. Knowles. We had the opportunity to interview him about Susan's treatment. In retrospect, he felt torn between his desire to maintain the alliance with Susan by accepting her decision about Grant and the pressure from staff in the hospital to take a firm stand. He felt he went against his own therapeutic intuition by setting such a rigid limit, but he felt compelled by his administrative position within the hospital to comply with the hospital guideline he helped to establish. Of course, he accepted her back into treatment after she was discharged, which attests to the strength of the relationship—that is, her willingness to return to see him as well as his to continue the therapy.

This incident also highlights the phenomena of splitting, when treatment team members are divided over how to approach the patient. It is extremely difficult to maintain a middle ground. Further, Susan's involvement with Grant did represent a loss of professional boundaries and mirrored the incestuous relationships in her family. It was important that staff was outraged and let Susan know they considered his behavior a breach of trust. Had he been currently employed, firing him would have been indicated. However, since Susan was an adult, nothing more could be done. Staff's extreme response was an example of assuming too much of the parental role and exercising inappropriate authority.

One other aspect of the residential treatment and her treatment with Dr. Knowles seemed to be lacking: an emphasis on Susan's education and training. Possibly because of her family's wealth, or because of her poor educational history, or because she was female, not much attention was placed on helping her develop skills and competence in hobbies or work-related areas. Such competence would have been important to her overall development and stability.

5

Kindness of Strangers...Sylvia

Whoever you are—I have always depended on the kindness of strangers.

Tennessee Williams, A Streetcar Named Desire

The Chestnut Lodge admitting doctor described Sylvia, a former actress, as an "attractive woman who is quite composed." Nothing in her manner suggested that she had spent most of her adult life in psychiatric hospitals. A veteran of 15 hospitalizations, treatment with electroconvulsive therapy (ECT), and numerous medications and psychotherapies, Sylvia began her odyssey as a professional inpatient at the age of 27. Over the next 9 years, Sylvia settled into a classic pattern of stable instability. Her admission to Chestnut Lodge was viewed as a last-chance effort to alter the downward spiral of her life.

HISTORY OF DISORDER

Sylvia's problems emerged most clearly when she left home to attend college. She was unable to adjust to college and changed schools twice during her first 2 years. In her third year and at her fourth school, Sylvia became despondent over a failed romance and overdosed for the first time. She dropped out of college and moved cross-country in search of an acting career.

At the age of 21, Sylvia met her husband-to-be, Billy, a moderately successful painter, 16 years her senior, who suffered from episodic depressions, binge drinking, and psychotic states. Sylvia dreamed he would make her famous. Billy, described as dapper and charming, left his troubled marriage and only son to live with Sylvia. Despite this, Sylvia became increasingly jealous of Billy's wife and slept with other men to assuage her insecurity. At the same time, and for the first and only period in her life, Sylvia worked steadily as a radio actress. After 3 years of living with Billy, Sylvia, hoping to bolster her self-esteem and stop her promiscuity, paid for Billy's divorce so they could marry.

A few months into the marriage, at age 24, Sylvia became anorgasmic, anxious, and phobic and burst into jealous tirades against Billy. Seeking help, she entered therapy with a female Jungian analyst but terminated after 6 months. She claimed she could not work with a woman and wanted a Freudian analysis, which was considered the superior treatment of the day.

During this "classical analysis," which lasted 18 months, Sylvia became pregnant. According to Billy, her analyst was against the pregnancy, but Sylvia waited too long for an abortion. Like her mother and grandmother, Sylvia suffered throughout her pregnancy and exhibited "violent hysterical outbursts" and phobias. After the birth of her son, James, Sylvia developed a postpartum depression. She became phobic of driving and had intrusive, recurring thoughts of killing her son.

Sylvia's analyst, apparently discouraged, told Billy he could no longer work with her, and Billy communicated this to Sylvia. Panicked by her symptoms and her analyst's hopelessness, she fled cross-country for her first private psychiatric hospitalization.

Over the next 9 years, Sylvia was in and out of the best private psychiatric hospitals in the United States for periods of a few days to 10 months. Her treatments included ECT, Thorazine, various sleeping medications, psychotherapy, and milieu therapies. She and Billy divorced and remarried during this time. She had one serious suicide attempt when she ingested arsenate of lead following a disastrous romance.

Her hospitalizations were usually precipitated by her alcoholism or a disruption in her relationship with Billy. When drinking, Sylvia screamed, broke dishes, and threatened suicide and bodily assault. She and Billy engaged in frequent, chaotic drunken fights characterized by vitriolic verbal abuse and, at times, physical aggression.

While in the hospital, Sylvia would rather quickly become a model patient, and her acute symptoms would remit. Between hospitalizations, Sylvia attempted to reestablish a home life with Billy and her son. She tried to cope through "obsessive hobby work and alcohol" and outpatient supportive treatment. She involved herself in the art community and learned pottery, for which she had considerable talent. Sylvia attempted to parent her son, but inevitably her own needs would become ascendant. When drinking, she was verbally abusive to him.

James was often left to the care of Sylvia's parents and caregivers they hired. Sylvia's hospitalization at Chestnut Lodge followed an overdose with sleeping pills prompted by a violent quarrel with Billy. There was "nothing in her outward behavior nor during this interview that would indicate a need for hospitalization." The doctor pointed this out to her, and she speculated that her training as an actress might have helped her to hide distress.

FAMILY AND DEVELOPMENTAL HISTORY

Mental disorders were pervasive in Sylvia's family. Her paternal grandfather was in and out of mental institutions for unspecified problems. Her maternal grandmother suffered a postpartum psychosis after the birth of Sylvia's mother. Similarly, Sylvia's mother developed a postpartum depression after her birth and, later, a psychotic depression. Sylvia's mother impressed the hospital staff as a "mean borderline psychotic . . . who controls her environment by outbursts of rage or complete withdrawal." Sylvia's father, a wealthy and successful farmer, was described as superficially charming and jovial. Underneath lay a "thrifty, hard-hearted, perfectionist who rules everyone with an iron hand, a ruthless, brilliant lone wolf who could become frankly psychotic."

Sylvia was conceived 20 years into her parents' marriage after father threatened to leave mother unless she consented to sexual relations; she had refused throughout their marriage. Sylvia later referred to herself as the glue that kept the marriage together. During and after the pregnancy, her mother was unable to care for Sylvia because of depression and anxiety. A "spinster nurse who was very rigid" served as surrogate mother. Later, a more kindly housekeeper assumed this role.

The only child of her older parents, Sylvia was raised on an isolated country estate with her nurse, a housekeeper, and her maternal grandmother as her primary companions. Sylvia was alternately grossly indulged or harshly deprived depending on the moods of her caregivers. Perceived as a sickly child, Sylvia was carried everywhere and did not walk until the age of 18 months. Father orchestrated her early social life by having children chauffeured to the estate for elaborate parties famous in the local town. Sylvia sat on the perimeter watching, having never learned how to play with other children. When Sylvia asked for a dollhouse, her father bought her such a large one that a later owner lived in it while remodeling his home. Concerned about Sylvia's schooling, her father hired a private teacher and began his own school.

Father, unwelcome in mother's bed, engaged a series of mistresses. Sylvia slept with mother until, when Sylvia was 8, her mother became agoraphobic and psychotically depressed and withdrew from family contact. Preoccupied with death, mother haunted the house reciting death poems. Suddenly terrified of the poorhouse, mother forbade Sylvia to buy clothes. Sylvia imagined puncturing herself with a needle to gain back her mother's attention. At age 9, after her grandmother's death, Sylvia developed a school phobia, which kept her home for several months.

Father turned to Sylvia at 13 as his confidante. The family chauffeur drove them on long trips through the countryside. Sylvia sat on father's lap as he caressed and kissed her and confided his love affairs, begging her forgiveness. She imagined herself Madame Pompadour or a back-alley mistress. Awakened and excited by these interludes, Sylvia sought one boy after another. Brief, passionate, albeit unconsummated, romances ensued and were ended by Sylvia's fear of being used for her family's money.

In high school, Sylvia developed skill as a singer and actress (her mother's youthful aspirations) and performed at school events often and successfully. She did well superficially and did not develop persistent problems until she went away to college.

COURSE IN TREATMENT AT CHESTNUT LODGE

The staff at Chestnut Lodge were dismayed with Sylvia's daunting treatment history. They were struck by her elusive quality, the absence of factual information regarding her history, and her vague and distracted manner. She was exquisitely sensitive; routine questions were interpreted as criticism, and silence was interpreted as neglect. Her emotions were intense but evanescent. She would weep profusely one minute and critique a film the next. Sylvia's verbal sophistication and knowledge of psychiatric terms dazzled just as her regal carriage and impeccable dress intimidated. She settled easily into the hospital milieu and was soon a model, if somewhat aloof, patient. Hopes were high that this time the tragic trajectory of Sylvia's life could be reversed.

When Sylvia first met her therapist, Dr. Willets, she expressed concern that he was too young and might not be strong enough for her. Dr. Willets also expressed discouragement when he heard that Sylvia had shown no improvement after 9 years of treatment. However, after meeting the still attractive and verbal Sylvia, who did not look or speak like a chronic patient, Dr. Willets felt "quite differently" and said, "I can work with her and like her."

Sylvia's depression lifted within the first week. She attributed her dramatic improvement to reading a newspaper story about the recovery of a leper after 20 years of ailment. She added, "Perhaps I also will have a chance."

Dr. Willets understood Sylvia's chief problem as her "extremely narcissistic and omnipotent fantasies." Sylvia wanted to be center stage in any social situation, and when this was challenged, she reacted first with rage, then with guilt, and finally with a desire to escape from the situation. Sylvia talked uninterruptedly throughout the hour and became extremely irritated whenever Dr. Willets made comments.

During the first month of treatment, Sylvia cried profusely, remarking that she was acting like a 3-year-old. She soon became critical of Dr. Willets for saying too much or too little. He observed that Sylvia did not seem to have any understanding as to why she was hospitalized. Dr. Willets expressed to the medical staff his concern over whether Sylvia could benefit from treatment, citing her poor response to prior treatment, her inability to live outside of the hospital, her shaky marriage, and her violent responses to the slightest rejections. Despite these reservations, Dr. Willets maintained hope primarily because of Sylvia's verbal abilities and sophisticated use of psychiatric language. As with Sylvia's prior therapists, her verbal intelligence and artistic abilities kept Dr. Willets engaged with her.

Dr. Willets was a recently graduated psychiatrist who was starting his analytic training. Despite his misgivings, he attempted a more traditional psychoanalytic approach. Sylvia was instructed to lie on the couch after 2 months and report all thoughts, emotions, bodily sensations, and dreams. She reported erotic dreams, talked "starkly" about her erotic feelings, and left sessions because of the "urgency of urination." As Sylvia declared her love and sexual desire for Dr. Willets, she would "work up to a near orgasm."

When Dr. Willets interpreted her behavior as defensive, Sylvia became enraged and missed sessions. When present, she characterized Dr. Willets as a cold and indifferent person like her mother. She taunted him with a lack of manliness. Following these sessions, Sylvia begged forgiveness and berated herself. She complained to her social worker that Dr. Willets was cold, inhuman, and distant. Sylvia complained to other staff that she felt fine on the days when she did not have analytic hours and tremendous anxiety when she did.

As in all other hospitalizations, Sylvia was described as a model patient within the social mileu. Sylvia became quickly involved with theatrical productions at Chestnut Lodge and had the lead in a hospital play. The director described Sylvia as very talented and a joy to work with despite her quick temper. Within 6 months, Sylvia had privileges to leave the grounds and was comanager of the patient-operated store and a member of the library committee and was active in the hospital-patient committee.

Despite her success, Sylvia was preoccupied with suicidal thoughts. She was concerned with pleasing everyone and felt she could not do anything right. When she did not receive explicit approval, she experienced frustration, became suicidal, and wanted to leave the hospital. During this time, Sylvia tearfully told her social worker that although she was tired of being isolated, she found getting close to people an emotionally disturbing experience.

During a case conference after 8 months of hospitalization, Dr. Willets described Sylvia as "extremely insecure . . . she wants to be in the limelight, but doesn't want to exercise any effort to achieve this." He saw Sylvia as beset by fears of success, autonomy, and intimacy and as coping with these anxieties with anger, alcohol, and suicide attempts. The treatment plan was to de-emphasize talk of her alcoholism or suicide attempts and to emphasize the underlying anger so she could gain greater conscious control.

Sylvia's mother became seriously ill at this time, and on her return from her mother's bedside Sylvia moved out of the hospital completely and began looking for a job. Billy began visiting her in her new apartment. Sylvia's mother died within a few weeks, and after the funeral, physical fights with Billy ensued. Dr. Willets described the couple's fights as "being drunk and trying to kill one another or anyone in their way." When Sylvia returned from her mother's funeral, she was rehospitalized. During her therapy hours, she was at first "emotionless" but then expressed suicidal wishes "to finish herself before being revenged."

During Billy's next visit, another fight erupted, the police were called, and he was taken to jail for one night. Dr. Willets noted, "With this kind of thing going on, therapy hours can only be used to deal with her emotions resulting from each episode. . . . she has not had the time or energy to do much work on understanding herself." Sylvia enlisted her friends to declare allegiance for or against Billy, and she would swing between plans for reunion or separation on the basis of their advice. Dr. Willets was frustrated that Sylvia could not benefit from his interpretations regarding her ambivalence about the marriage. She gave "lip service to the fact that the problem rested with herself" and her "capacity to love" while holding on to her belief that a decision to stay or go was really the heart of the matter. The therapy hours were filled with detailed descriptions of her friends' advice, which Dr. Willets felt was Sylvia's resistance to exploring her behaviors and responsibilities in the marital dynamics.

Sylvia, now spending more time in the community, sought and secured a leading part in a local play. With her acceptance of the role, therapy hours focused on Sylvia's fear of success and failure and her need to be special. Sylvia wondered if her years of hospitalization served as a protection against competition with normal people, as she always felt superior to her hospital mates. It was this kind of comment that confused her therapist into thinking she had a capacity for greater self-awareness.

Toward the end of her second year at Chestnut Lodge, Sylvia was offered two acting jobs and accepted one as a supporting player. Sylvia envied the leading lady and ruminated over how much better she could do in the part. When Dr. Willets attempted to keep her focused on the theme of competition, Sylvia objected, saying, "You are just like my mother . . . when you push your ideas on me."

Sylvia's father, now in his eighties, visited Chestnut Lodge. Although he provided complete financial support for Sylvia and her son and was available for phone calls, this was his only reported visit throughout her numerous hospitalizations. During this brief visit, the narcissistic features of his personality were evident. He dominated the conversation. He expounded on his self-cure of tongue cancer through dietary means, although doctors recommended surgery. The social worker stated, "He doesn't listen to the other person and doesn't care who is listening; he talks for himself."

Dr. Willets attempted to organize a presentation on Sylvia's treatment but felt unable. He explained, "There really is too much to organize . . . it's too much material to present. . . . I have very little impression of what is under the facade that she presents to her public. I'm still at sea about what goes on. . . . [She] mentions a topic and then branches off into something else and very rarely follows-through with intent to discover something useful about her behavior that could be changed."

Sylvia remained an outpatient for another year. Billy entered treatment in another city and accepted a well-paying job requiring considerable travel. Billy's success frightened Sylvia, and she wondered if it was a prelude to his deserting her. She complained of loneliness and considered an affair. Her phobia of driving returned, causing further isolation, and she experienced increased anxiety and somatic complaints. As a way to fill her lonely days, Sylvia accepted a part-time job as a salesperson.

At midyear she accepted a part in a new play, and Billy visited to provide support. During another drinking bout, they got into an argument and discussed divorce. Sylvia called the hospital, intoxicated and upset, and was advised to admit herself overnight. At the hospital, Sylvia cried that she did not want to live and that no one cared, and she pleaded with staff to hold her hand and help her. Her tears suddenly converted to anger. Sylvia cursed the nurse and threw a glass of milk across the desk. Just as suddenly Sylvia organized herself and said, "I'm acting again. I'm very dramatic." She requested sedation, but when this was denied, Sylvia, again angry, threatened to wreck the dayroom stating, "I came here to get some rest before my next role. . . . Oh! you people don't know what it is to create something!" Sylvia grabbed and hugged the nurse following this outburst and assured her she would try to get some sleep.

Sylvia transitioned to full outpatient status over the next 2 months as she maintained her apartment, held a part-time sales job, and continued theater work. Staff reported that Sylvia was getting along better with her son and her father and had improved social contact. Dr. Willets felt that Sylvia had "improved a great deal"; she was no longer chronically depressed, did not resort constantly to self-destructiveness, rarely drank by herself to intoxication, and was more positive toward life. Ever hopeful, he predicted that with further treatment, Sylvia's "capacity to relate to people would increase and she would be more able to realize her potentialities and make use of them."

Sylvia continued with Dr. Willets in private treatment for three more years. The summaries of the treatment suggest that the up-and-down course of the treatment was similar to that of her previous treatment, although Sylvia was able to remain outside of the hospital.

One treatment segment bears noting because it supports the injurious nature of Sylvia's relationship with her father. Sylvia had recalled their physical closeness when she was 13 years of age. Dr. Willets suggested that the relationship was incestuous. Sylvia responded with a brief conversion reaction. Her legs became paralyzed as she recalled heart-to-heart talks with her father as he held her on his lap and confided sexual experiences with his many mistresses while begging her forgiveness. In the retelling of these experiences, she was flooded with emotions she barely understood. Sylvia may also have repeated a similar incestuous-like relationship with her son. At age 14, he told her he wanted to have sexual relations with her. He, too, was now in psychiatric treatment.

When the treatment ended, Sylvia planned to reunite with her husband in another state because they each found the other had "mellowed." Their son, who was now in a preparatory boarding school, also urged them to try to live together. Sylvia hoped to take up her acting career even though she was by now 41 and had not pursued it in 3 years. Her continued difficulties were foreshadowed by her often-spoken remark to Dr. Willets, "I'm glue, but no body."

FOLLOW-UP TWENTY YEARS LATER

Follow-up was conducted 20 years after termination of private treatment with Dr. Willets. Sylvia had died recently, at the age of 59, of cancer. Dr. Leonard, her last therapist, provided the follow-up information.

Although Sylvia told Dr. Leonard that she had never liked Dr. Willets because he was too cold, she felt that she had made good progress while in therapy with him. In contrast to his comments in the last treatment summary, Dr. Willets, in response to the follow-up questionnaire, rated Sylvia's functioning at discharge as "little to no improvement."

After leaving Chestnut Lodge, Sylvia lived with Billy until his death 6 years later. She saw a psychiatrist at least twice a week throughout and was hospitalized every 3–4 months for depression, drinking, and suicide attempts. When Billy died, Sylvia moved back to her family home, where she remained for 4 years with her son until he married. She saw a psychiatrist there once a week, continued drinking, and "ate Triavils (a combination antidepressant and antipsychotic medication) like peanuts."

Without the support of her father, Billy, or her son, Sylvia spiraled further into chronic alcoholism and prescription drug addiction. Ten years after her discharge from Chestnut Lodge, Sylvia, at age 51, returned for treatment of addiction to the site of her first hospitalization. She stated that she planned to remain in or near the hospital for the rest of her life, which she did.

At this admission, she met Dr. Leonard, her last therapist, and she was given a diagnosis of borderline personality disorder with "strong infantile and hysterical features." Dr. Leonard also diagnosed "alcoholic encephalopathy" on the basis of Sylvia's slurred speech, neuromuscular twitching of her extremities, and mild memory impairment. The long-term consequences of alcoholism had taken their toll. Unable to manage her own affairs, Sylvia was placed on conservatorship.

Sylvia saw Dr. Leonard three times a week and was maintained regularly on Thorazine and sporadically on Sinequan, Valium, and chloral hydrate. Lithium was prescribed for a 6-month period but was discontinued for unknown reasons. Dr. Leonard attempted to "wean her from Valium," but she "reacted with rage . . . as though we were depriving her of mother's breast." Other attempts to reduce her drug intake were met with abuse of over-the-counter drugs and suicide threats. Sylvia explained she "would go crazy without some props or chemical means of controlling herself."

Dr. Leonard described her treatment course as one of a "classic, intense, inpatient career of a borderline patient with a positive erotic transference to the therapist and split-off negative transference onto the staff." In therapy, he described Sylvia as a professional patient with intellectual insight.

Sylvia typifies what we would now characterize as a dually diagnosed revolving-door patient who is hospitalized repeatedly for suicide attempts and alcohol detoxification. Most of the hospitalizations occurred around Dr. Leonard's vacation, a fight with her son, or loss of a live-in companion. Sylvia's physical health also continued to deteriorate, requiring lengthy hospital stays.

As before, Sylvia's life pattern was consistently unstable. After initial detoxification and stabilization in the hospital, she rented an apartment, obtained her driver's license, and bought a car. She joined Alcoholics Anonymous and became active in the patient council. As Sylvia prepared to move into an apartment, she arranged for a maid from her hometown to come live with her. Initially, she was active socially and involved herself in a local play. Her "improvements" would invariably be followed by a crisis characterized by depression, increased drinking, suicidal feelings, and another hospitalization. This pattern continued until her death.

Between hospitalizations, Sylvia bought a house that she furnished extensively with antiques, made pottery that was exhibited at a local gallery, and attempted various volunteer jobs such as tutoring adolescents. Without friends, Sylvia's only ongoing relationships were with hired professionals: her therapist, conservator, and lawyer. Her extreme sensitivity colored all of her interactions, and she perceived insult and injury in most encounters. Sylvia was unable to maintain a consistent tie with live-in hired companions. The daily contact inevitably led to disappointment and either dismissal by her or resignation by them. Although she could put forward an acceptable and entertaining social facade for brief periods, she became enraged or depleted by longer-term or more intense interpersonal involvements.

Typical of this pattern, Sylvia dated on only two occasions. She had intercourse with the first man and, when she developed an infection, broke off the relationship. The second man she dismissed quickly when she felt criticized.

Her son, daughter-in-law, and grandchildren were Sylvia's sole remaining family. She visited them on several occasions and sent the children lavish presents "to make up for what she didn't do for her son." These relationships, too, ended bitterly. During her final visit, Sylvia brought suitcases full of painting and pottery supplies and tried to promote her grandchildren into becoming artists. Her daughter-in-law objected, and they quarreled. Sylvia, rebuffed, began drinking and unleashed a torrent of vicious criticism. Intoxicated, she called her conservator, threatened suicide, and returned home. This was apparently Sylvia's last contact with her son. When she asked to have him notified of her terminal illness, he failed to respond.

Sylvia's health deteriorated further. Cognitively, she became increasingly vulnerable to paranoid states. When alone at night, Sylvia feared the house was haunted by her mother. She could smell her mother's perfume and saw her in a rocking chair. Sylvia periodically registered into a nearby hotel to avoid these experiences and asked her conservator to visit and check out the house.

In his discharge summary, Dr. Leonard described the course of treatment in fair detail. Like all of Sylvia's therapists before him, he was surprised at first with how sharp, intelligent, and vivacious Sylvia was. She enjoyed talking about politics, art, and dramatics and was "delightful" at these times. However, if Dr. Leonard tried to share in the conversation with her, Sylvia would accuse him of invading her privacy and ruining her presentation. Sylvia had to be center stage.

The therapy was full of talk about her dynamics and the "meaning" of their relationship. Nevertheless, Dr. Leonard acknowledged that Sylvia's intellectual insight did not contribute to any change in feeling or behavior and that she perceived therapy as "a means of gratification." For example, Sylvia once overdosed while he was away on vacation despite the fact that "they had discussed the meaning of his absence in great detail."

His therapeutic optimism still persisted as he focused on her improvements and "rapid" recoveries from numerous suicide attempts and hospitalizations. He seemed heartened when Sylvia talked about reducing her therapy visits to twice a week and encouraged her when she decided to dismiss her nighttime live-in companion. At the same time, Dr. Leonard recognized her need for continuous containment. He attended Sylvia's art showings with his wife and accepted numerous nighttime phone calls and long-distance crisis calls. He drove to Sylvia's house when she called him in a panic state, and he served as case manager coordinating Sylvia's care by physicians, live-in caregivers, and conservator.

Toward the end of her life, Sylvia could still rally even though in failing physical and mental health. She wrote a moving speech for the dedication ceremony of a new building at the hospital. She bought a kiln, made her own ceramic pieces, and planned remodeling work on her house. Six months before Sylvia's death, in the midst of radiation therapy, she delivered her speech for the dedication ceremony. When asked for permission to have her speech published in the hospital newspaper, Sylvia proudly agreed. This brief triumph was short-lived when she was told the paper's policy was to not use names so as to protect patient confidentiality. Sylvia, outraged, protested to the hospital staff and administrators. She felt her one worthwhile contribution would go unrecognized. A compromise was reached; her speech was published with her initials.

Sylvia fought one last battle. She had hoped that one of the hospital aides could care for her at night but was told it was against hospital policy. Sylvia fell back on her usual coping style and began drinking and threatening suicide. Dr. Leonard suggested that the aide resign her position in the hospital and spend evenings with Sylvia during the last months of her life. With this accommodation, Sylvia "seemed to settle down, was busy, and active in her hobbies."

She finished the remodeling of her house, which "gave her great pleasure." When Sylvia learned that the cancer had spread, Dr. Leonard wrote, she "accepted the fact of her death, made funeral arrangements and a new will, leaving all of her personal belongings to the hospital aide." She died peacefully at home.

DISCUSSION OF ETIOLOGY AND OUTCOME OF DISORDER

We judged Sylvia's disorder to be severe and her outcome to be moderately poor. She had severe genetic and biological vulnerabilities in interaction with moderate child maltreatment and adverse life events.

Etiology

Biological and Environmental Risk Factors

Severe mental illnesses in the form of psychotic level disorders were present in both maternal and paternal grandparents. Sylvia's mother suffered from episodic psychotic depressions in interaction with a severe borderline disorder. Sylvia's father appeared to have a severe narcissistic personality disorder but was intact enough to achieve professional success.

Sylvia experienced cumulative biparental neglect of her emotional needs and a malignant form of parental overprotectiveness and indulgence. Both parents grossly disregarded her childhood needs and used her as a puppetlike extension of themselves. As we often see in narcissistic disorders, the parents were overly attentive to aspects of Sylvia's functioning that met their needs such as her attractiveness and acting ability.

Sylvia's mother's behaviors were unpredictable (stably unstable) and alternated among withdrawal, rage, overindulgence, overprotectiveness, hostile intrusiveness, and cruelty. Mother let Sylvia sleep in her bed until the age of 8 and then abruptly threw her out when mother was acutely depressed. Mother's communications when depressed were psychotic—for example, quoting poems for the dying and refusing to buy clothes for fear of poverty despite the family's wealth. Both parents created and reinforced Sylvia's expectation of special treatment. Mother demanded that Sylvia be given the lead in a school play, and father ordered the town's children to play with her. Father was overindulgent, seductive, and overstimulating and parentified Sylvia. His use of the 13-year-old Sylvia as confessor/confidante for his sexual liaisons revealed total unawareness of a child's needs. That he sexually used and abused Sylvia is likely.

Also, Sylvia witnessed a marriage without warmth, affection, or communication. She carried the additional burden of being the "glue" that kept the parent's marriage together. Finally, the family was extremely isolated from the local community. The grandmother who lived with Sylvia early in her life was very disturbed, and the live-in housekeeper was apparently cold and rigid. There did not appear to be any other extended family or friends who could lend balance and support.

Protective Factors

The family's wealth was a protective factor. Without it, Sylvia may have ended up homeless or even have died earlier from suicide or the effects of alcoholism. The support system it paid for enabled Sylvia to be continuously reclaimed from the brink of disaster and to function at her best when stable. Without her trust fund, she might have become homeless, because she would have been unable to tolerate the conditions and requirements in residential facilities. She also might have died younger from a successful, albeit accidental, suicide attempt or from cirrhosis of the liver.

Another factor was Sylvia's intrinsic abilities and attributes: her attractiveness, intelligence, and verbal and artistic ability. Also, she had developed the capacity for concentrated attention and self-discipline when stable. Employing these abilities, she had a capacity to engage others. As long as she was admired without any expectation of mutuality, the relationship could continue. These personal qualities also enabled Sylvia to maintain a relationship with a therapist. Within the safety of the therapeutic relationship, she was the actress and the therapist was the admiring audience.

Unlike Susan's father (see Chapter 4), Sylvia's father appeared to enjoy continued success in his profession. The family lived in the same place until the parents' death. This, too, provided Sylvia with a stable, albeit disturbed, home base while her parents were alive and enabled her to develop greater skills in daily living and to pursue an education and hobbies.

Outcome

Sylvia struggled almost continuously from a disorganized attachment mode and resultant behavioral collapse in response to separation and narcissistic injury. She remained unable to regulate her emotions and behavior in response to disruptions in her attachment to others. Her cognitive functioning deteriorated as a consequence of alcoholism. Although no real development took place, Sylvia's disorder could be contained by the continuous prosthesis of her therapeutic community. She was at her most stable in a detached attachment mode maintained through aloofness and an "as if" quality of superiority. In this attachment mode, she could maintain involvement in a nonmutual relationship with a benign caregiver such as her therapist, lawyer, and live-in aide and with people in the town who could admire her from afar as a "local artist."

Cognitive Dysfunction

Paranoid ideation.   As early as junior high school, Sylvia suspected that peers were out to use her to get at her family money. Her paranoia was expressed throughout her life as extreme sensitivity to insult or deprivation. She took offense easily and often. Paranoia sparked her jealous tirades toward her husband and anger toward therapists and caregivers. The paranoia continued until her death.

Sylvia exhibited black-and-white thinking, especially in relationship to others, who were perceived as all good or all bad. She manifested an overvalued idea about her own specialness that directed much of her behavior. One hospital report described a quality of "diffuse distractiveness" that alluded to an inability to maintain coherent lines of thought. Sylvia bounced from idea to idea.

Although Sylvia was intermittently diagnosed as having schizophrenia because of the degree of disorganization prior to hospital admissions, there were no reports of psychotic-like thinking until late in her life. At that time, and probably related to cognitive deterioration associated with alcoholism and Sylvia's deep isolation, she developed a sense that her mother was haunting her house. This vision was accompanied with olfactory illusions of mother's perfume and visual illusions of her mother rocking in a chair. This vision, rather than comforting Sylvia, frightened her and serves as a poignant testimony to how early trauma persists. Also, the record mentions memory difficulty and slurred speech, perhaps related to alcoholism and possible undiagnosed small strokes.

Dissociation. There was mention of dissociation, which preceded her angry outbursts in earlier hospital records, but no explicit report of such episodes occurred while Sylvia was at Chestnut Lodge. However, dissociation is suggested in her unusual composure, aloofness, and "as if" quality.

Emotional Regulation

Affective instability. Sylvia's hospital discharge summary captured her mood lability as follows: "[Sylvia] has a very colorful, intensive emotional life which is markedly lacking in stability and can easily turn into emotional dullness or over-emotionalism and outbursts of anger." She also appeared to experience acute panic states and, when relationships were disrupted, a pervasive and debilitating anxiety. Sylvia, like her mother and grandmother before her, also had depressive episodes, usually characterized by extreme agitation. All her affective problems were aggravated by substance dependence, abuse of prescription medications, and the cycle of addiction and detoxification.

Intense anger or lack of control of anger. Records suggested that Sylvia's anger, sparked by mistrust of others' motives and exquisite sensitivity to perceived slight or criticism, expressed itself in high school through a demeaning and devaluing style of "dropping" friends and boyfriends. The case depiction of Sylvia's mother as "controlling her environment through outbursts of rage or complete withdrawal" could also have been written about Sylvia. Her first psychiatrist described "violent hysterical outbursts." Sylvia erupted into jealous tirades and, when under the influence of alcohol or drugs, assaulted her husband. Her frequent temper tantrums in response to perceived insult and deprivation alienated everyone except her therapists.

Assaultive behavior appeared confined to the marital relationship; there were no reports of physical violence after the death of Sylvia's husband. In contrast, the intensity of Sylvia's demeaning anger and its frequent verbal display appeared constant over the course of her lifetime. The damaging effects of Sylvia's anger on her life were evident in her estrangement from her son and grandchildren, her inability to keep friendships, and her inability to retain a live-in housekeeper.

Behavioral Regulation

Impulsive/compulsive use of pleasurable behaviors. Sylvia was reported to be promiscuous prior to her marriage to Billy, but her behavior functioned as a means to tolerate his marriage and seek revenge. She would also "neck openly with house guests" in front of Billy to torture him when concerned about his alleged infidelity. Her impulsive behavior was often a response to feeling injured by Billy and a means of retaliating.

Sylvia's substance use was addictive rather than impulsive. She exhibited impulsivity under the influence of alcohol and other drugs. Sylvia's life highlights the vulnerability that individuals with severe borderline or narcissistic disorders have toward substance dependence and the complications it creates in the course of their disorder.

Alcohol and drugs aggravated Sylvia's extremely fragile psychological system, multiplied her interpersonal failures, and contributed to suicidal behavior, violence, serious health problems, and cognitive impairment. Sylvia believed "she would go crazy without some props or chemical means of controlling herself." She "ate Triavil like peanuts," reacted with rage when an attempt was made to wean her from Valium, and resorted to abuse of over-the-counter drugs. Sylvia was clearly frantic at the thought of being deprived of a substance to alter or modulate her normally empty and dysphoric state. Alcohol and other drugs had replaced sustaining relationships to a large extent.

Suicidal/self-mutilative behavior. At the age of 8, Sylvia imagined puncturing herself with a needle as a means of gaining mother's attention but never reported actually cutting herself. Sylvia's first overdose, in her late teens, occurred in response to a failed romance. This began a pattern of preoccupation with suicide and suicide attempts throughout her life.

During the follow-up period, Sylvia's suicide threats and attempts escalated. She overdosed in response to any perceived abandonment, such as Dr. Leonard's vacations, fights with her son, and the loss of live-in companions. It is difficult to evaluate whether Sylvia's overdoses were an expression of a serious intent to die or the accidental result of an overuse of alcohol and drugs when her already insecure attachments were further threatened. Her most serious attempt occurred in the last 2 years of her life, when she cut her radial artery. The precipitant to this attempt was not mentioned, but we speculate it, too, was related to perceived narcissistic injury and abandonment in combination with her increased disinhibition and carelessness related to advanced alcoholism.

Abandonment fears. As described in the previous section, Sylvia responded to being alone with increased drinking, suicide attempts, and behavioral disorganization. She relied on hospital staff as her extended family and functioned best within the structure and support of the hospital or in close proximity to it.

Sylvia had minimal internal resources and was without a capacity for evocative memory, and when she was left alone, her adaptive behavioral strategies crumbled. Sylvia's life illustrates the experience of abandonment for BPD patients. When significant others are not present, the relationship truly disappears. Sylvia was once again a helpless and panicked toddler randomly seeking solace through alcohol and attempting to restore control through temper tantrums.

Unstable Intense Relationships

Dr. Simpson, Sylvia's earliest psychotherapist, noted that Sylvia was searching for an all-understanding figure and expressed intense rage if her expectations were not met. Sylvia acknowledged that she was chronically disappointed in others. She expressed her disappointment with therapists through demeaning comments, temper outbursts, and missed sessions. In her marriage, Sylvia exhibited her extreme sensitivity through the intensity of her reactions to Billy. She characteristically overdosed or became drunk and violent or unable to function when without him.

Sylvia had one affair while in the hospital during a separation from Billy. It was so disturbing that Sylvia made a nearly lethal suicide attempt following its end. Her doctor wrote that relationships depleted her and she needed to withdraw. Sylvia was incapable either of forming friendships or of maintaining a working relationship with companions. Her behavior toward her son and his family was so toxic that he refused all contact even when Sylvia was dying.

Despite its stormy course, Sylvia maintained her marriage until Billy's death. This seemed related to both partners being unable to function without each other. Billy may also have been bound to her as his sole means of financial support. Sylvia could maintain only a relatively stable long-term relationship with people paid to be tolerant and accepting—namely, therapists and lawyers. She even had difficulty with paid companions, probably because of the constant physical proximity that eventually required some mutuality.

Identity Disturbance

Sylvia's self-image fluctuated from "a person alone in a dark forest . . . [who] had a few fragile controls above a bottomless sea of dark illness" to a grandiose self who believed that she had special talents and deserved special treatment. Sylvia's gender and sexual identity were stably feminine and heterosexual. However, the records suggest that Sylvia was unable to enjoy sexual relations. She did not have the capacity for an intimate and loving sexual relationship. Also, even the most basic sexual involvement probably placed too great a demand for mutuality on her and further disorganized her. For much of her adult life, Sylvia held an identity as a married woman and a mother. Despite her failure in these roles, this identity provided a structure to her life. She apparently was able to organize, decorate, and maintain a home and attend to minimal daily chores.

Sylvia was able to complete high school and some college and to pursue special training as an actress. She did have talent and artistic ability. This enabled her to work until her disorder and substance abuse consumed her energies. Although unable to sustain work beyond her twenties, Sylvia continued to perform episodically in amateur theater and, when this became too stressful, to create ceramic pieces. She had talent for decorating and was knowledgeable about antiques, and she had a flair for dress and presentation. She also was well read and a lively conversationalist.

Sylvia maintained her avocation as an artist, which, combined with her presentation of self, provided her with a niche within the community as well as a source of enjoyment. Her avocation and interest in the arts appeared to sustain her during more stable periods of functioning. This niche also afforded Sylvia a modicum of the special treatment for which she yearned.

DISCUSSION OF TREATMENT

Comparison With Current Treatments

Sylvia typifies the challenge of treating patients with co-occurring substance abuse and dependence, mood disorders, anxiety disorders, and BPD with prominent narcissistic features. Dr. Leonard's comment that weaning her from Valium was like depriving her of mother's breast was more prescient than he knew. Sylvia's comment that she would go crazy without a chemical prop was equally perceptive. The challenge then, as today, with patients who experience such intense emotional emptiness or extreme anxiety and dysphoria when alone is how to provide pharmacological intervention without compounding the addiction.

Although the single most destructive feature in her course, Sylvia's addiction was minimized throughout her treatment probably because of a much greater public tolerance for alcohol abuse in the late 1950s and early 1960s and the then-prevailing belief that psychotherapy could treat alcoholism. Thus, the alcoholism was understood as a symptom and not a separate disorder in need of its own treatment. Only in the last years of Sylvia's life was involvement with Alcoholics Anonymous mentioned.

However, even today, treatment options are limited for patients with dual disorders, and a double stigma is attached. Also, patients who have narcissistic features often find group self-help approaches demeaning and refuse to attend. Today, however, there is an increased likelihood that her vulnerability to addiction would be identified sooner and there would be a concerted focus of treatment, through either an integrated treatment program or parallel involvement in psychiatric treatment and self-help groups. Abstinence would be advised and Antabuse (disulfiram) or naltrexone would be considered. Medications now available might be more effective in treating her mood instability, anxiety, and depression, which might assist with abstinence from alcohol and greater overall affective stability.

Sylvia's treatment toward the end of her life was optimal in many respects and would continue to serve as a good standard of care. Today, she might still be a revolving-door patient in and out of private inpatient drug detoxification and rehabilitation centers and psychiatric hospitals, although stays at the latter would be much briefer. Her wealth would continue to serve as a protective factor, in that she could afford to pay for private care. This care would include working with a psychotherapist to provide a continuous supportive therapeutic relationship, with the goal of maintaining function, reducing self-destructive behaviors, and improving quality of life, and a psychiatrist for psychopharmacological treatment.

Therapeutic Factors

Sylvia, too, benefited primarily from the asylum and village functions provided at Chestnut Lodge. She always functioned best within the structure of the hospital. She had people around, but intimacy was not required. She could even work successfully within the sheltered workshop of the residential setting. Similarly, the structure provided by the psychoanalytic framework served a prosthetic function for her. She had an identity as a psychiatric patient, a weekly schedule, and a parental figure interested in her. With this structure, she could maintain a detached attachment that was her most stable.

During the last 10 years of her life, her wealth enabled her to design her own mental health support system based on an assertive case management model. Her team consisted of Dr. Leonard, her case manager/therapist/psychiatrist, who even made home visits; a conservator; her AA group; a series of live-in case aides, who oversaw her care; and access to a nearby hospital. With this village surrounding her, she could be semiproductive, doing some volunteer work and making pottery. However, even with this level of support, she was unable to sustain steady functioning or stay abstinent from alcohol.

Countertherapeutic Factors

Sylvia's intelligence, verbal fluency, and artistic talent engendered unrealistic expectations regarding her capacity for improvement. Although the structure of psychoanalytic therapy may have been helpful, the interpersonal and cognitive demands were too great and triggered behavioral disorganization. Interpretations were consistently experienced as intrusions and narcissistic assaults, and the expectation of intimacy that psychotherapy implies placed too great a strain on her slim resources. We wondered if a self psychologically based approach might have been more helpful if begun early in her treatment. An earlier and greater appreciation of the severity of her narcissistic vulnerability might have prompted a more effective strategy. However, before her hospitalization at Chestnut Lodge and during another residential treatment, she engaged in a highly supportive psychotherapy. The treatment plan was switched to psychoanalysis because she had not improved.

An overestimation of the BPD patient's ability to incorporate interpretations and develop insight continues to be a common mistake made by therapists. Even Dr. Leonard, who, in our estimation, was the best possible psychiatrist and therapist for Sylvia and intuitively did what was best for her, persisted in thinking that she could benefit from insight. He could not fully understand how completely their relationship disappeared in his absence. The developmental damage, in conjunction with the underlying biological vulnerability, occurred too early and was too extensive and persistent.

Therapist Struggles

Sylvia typifies the challenge therapists face in the assessment of intelligent and talented patients with severe BPD. It is difficult to fully understand how poorly organized their attachment models are and how inadequate the cognitive structure is on which to build. It is hard to grasp the extent of cognitive disorganization wrought by poorly integrated attachment modes and information-processing deficits. There persists a belief that with "enough" therapy or the "right" therapy these patients can gain insight and improve. Like Dr. Willets, the therapist strains to make sense and organize the patient's voluminous and rambling or spare and vague material, not realizing that patients with severe personality disorders are unable to organize the material and find meaning.

Sylvia's case also highlights the importance of the North American overemphasis on individuality, autonomy, and progress. Such overemphasis may interfere with our ability to accept the importance of fostering a stable attachment to the mental health and social service system for the severely disabled patient. The persistent pressure to become autonomous placed on patients like Sylvia often dooms them to repeated failure.

Sylvia's case teaches humility and the importance of tempering therapeutic zeal with realism. Aspects of her treatment aggravated or worsened her condition, and effective medications were not available. However, even if these aspects had been corrected, Sylvia would still represent among the most challenging patients in our field. Her life also makes a powerful statement about the importance of providing asylum and a village through our mental health and social service systems. A good alternative to the state hospital system and private long-term residential hospitals like Chestnut Lodge still does not exist.

6

Wild at Heart...Wendy

Humpty Dumpty sat on a wall
Humpty Dumpty had a great fall
Threescore men and threescore more
Couldn't put Humpty Dumpty as he was before.

Nursery rhyme

Everything was a stimulus around me and I was the response.

Patient quote

Wild at heart and weird on top.

David Lynch

Wendy, described at admission to Chestnut Lodge in the late 1950s as a winning and coy 17-year-old, was transferred from another private psychiatric hospital after attempting to choke her latest therapist. Hospitalized the prior 2 years for cutting herself and assaulting others, Wendy had exhausted numerous therapists and defeated all treatment interventions. None of the standard treatments of the day, including Thorazine, restraints, seclusion, hydrotherapy, and hypnosis, appeared to effect any change. Having fired one doctor after another, Wendy set personnel one against the other and displayed Machiavellian genius for humiliating staff around sensitive areas. In defeat, the institution recommended a transfer to Chestnut Lodge.

HISTORY OF DISORDER

Wendy exhibited behavioral problems in grade school through temper tantrums and holding her breath when upset. By the age of 10, she was cutting herself in response to anger and humiliation. Although clearly in need of help earlier, she first received psychiatric attention around age 14 when her father arranged for her placement in a home for emotionally disturbed children. On entering the home, Wendy purposefully cut her leg. The wound became infected, and her leg was put in traction. The wrong splint was used, and she developed gangrene in her heel. When in the splint, Wendy also developed appendicitis. After surgery for both conditions, a spur was found on her heel requiring further surgery. Once recuperated, and while playing tennis, she jumped across the net, fell, and broke her wrist. Her father visited and accused her of breaking it on purpose. In response, she cut the bottoms of her feet to resemble blisters. After only 2 months in the home, the headmistress informed Wendy's father that her staff was incapable of providing further care. As such, Wendy's first psychiatric hospitalization was arranged, and she stayed off and on at that hospital for the next 3 years, until another exhausted staff recommended transfer to Chestnut Lodge.

FAMILY HISTORY

Although trained as an engineer, Wendy's father never worked because Wendy's mother demanded that he stay home with her. Father suffered from alcoholism, and when drinking, he was physically and emotionally abusive to his wife and children. There was also a suggestion from this record that his thinking was unusual.

Mother, described as lovely and elegant, came from an extremely wealthy family. The family money, generated by her great-grandfather, left subsequent generations free from work. Mother appeared to suffer from a severe personality disorder, psychotic depressions, and alcoholism.

The parents lived on a huge estate isolated from the community. Their married life was chaotic and characterized by alcoholic bouts, physical fights, and sexual promiscuity with others. They had three children within 5 years, and what fragile family stability existed collapsed when father was stationed overseas during World War II for 3 years. While father was gone, Wendy's mother was unable to parent the children, and they were left to fend for themselves, except for the physical caregiving provided by a series of housekeepers and aides. A fourth child was born after father's return. What family life existed was completely destroyed by mother's death in a fire that was triggered by a lit cigarette that she held while intoxicated and asleep in her bed. Wendy was 13.

Wendy was the third of four siblings. Wendy's sister, Carrie, was 3 years older and described as the only one of the four children able to live independently as an adult. Although she struggled with depression and was periodically in outpatient therapy and taking antidepressant medication, Carrie was able to maintain her role as homemaker and mother. Wendy's brother Eric, 2 years older, was severely emotionally disturbed as a child. Despite considerable treatment and numerous hospitalizations, he committed suicide in his mid-thirties. He had suffered for many years with severe depression, alcoholism, and ego-dystonic homosexuality. At the time of his death, he was living in a rooming house, unemployed. Andy, 7 years younger than Wendy, was described as "like an animal." He tortured animals, set fires, and was completely unsocialized. As an adult, he was hospitalized in a long-term treatment facility for alcoholism and antisocial personality disorder.

DEVELOPMENTAL HISTORY

Wendy was born while her father was on active duty overseas. When Wendy was 2 months old, mother wrote a final notation in Wendy's birthday book, "I see no reason to go on without my husband," and retreated into alcohol and to her bed. Wendy and her older brother and sister were cared for by nursemaids. When father returned home, he found the children neglected and the house in disarray. Wendy recoiled from her father, and he found it difficult to establish a relationship with her. At 3 years of age, Wendy stormed through the house screaming and breaking things. She also held her breath episodically until she turned blue.

Within months of father's return, both parents drank late into the night and provoked each other with talk of sexual liaisons. Their bitter, drunken fights often ended in bloodshed. When father was out of the home, mother retreated to her bedroom and was attended by a private nurse. She had numerous somatic complaints and frightened her children with talk of terminal illness.

Beginning at age 4, Wendy would be sent away to camp while her parents traveled. During her stays at camp, Wendy developed a variety of illnesses and was accident prone. At home, Wendy was cared for by Bessie, who had been hired as a cook but served as a surrogate parent. She called the doctor when the children were ill and signed report cards.

Unfortunately, she, too, was alcoholic, and Wendy often accompanied Bessie to her favorite bar.

In grade school, Wendy managed to get Bs and Cs and scored in the average to above-average range on achievement tests. Wendy maintained her standing in class until mother's death, when she had to repeat the eighth grade. Behavioral problems in the classroom appeared early, as Wendy had temper outbursts and continued to hold her breath when upset.

After school, Wendy played with animals on the family farm. Wendy's sole human companion and playmate was her older brother, Eric. Eric's play took the form of strangling birds to the edge of death and then attempting resuscitation. He set fires compulsively and broke into neighboring houses. Neighboring families forbade their children to play with Wendy.

Wendy experienced her mother as physically and emotionally unavailable, as she was often locked in her bedroom. When present, mother was disapproving, mean, and frightening. Father, although more present, was often drunk and subjected Wendy and her brothers to cruel unpredictable and vicious physical abuse and constant criticism. The record states, without providing further detail, that he was sexually inappropriate with Wendy and that mother was sexually seductive with her sons. Only the eldest daughter, raised during the only stable period in the parents' marital life, was spared the worst of the parent's behavior.

By age 10, Wendy was cutting herself in response to feelings of anger or humiliation. As she approached puberty, father's friends made sexual advances toward her at drunken parties at the compound. The records indicated that mother turned to the adolescent Eric for sexual comfort and would take him to her bed.

Mother's death ended what little remained of a family structure. Father, alone, began a nightly ritual of coming to Wendy's room and falling asleep drunk on top of her. The reports did not specify if there was actual sexual involvement. Her sister married, and Eric left for boarding school. Mother had cut father out of her will and left all to the children. Father contested but lost. The courts did not trust Wendy's father or sister and placed her in the custody of her new brother-in-law.

Wendy's behavior became increasingly disorganized and unmanageable after her mother's funeral. She rampaged throughout the house breaking furniture, refused to attend school, and assaulted playmates. Father, heir to a bankrupt company and barely functional himself, arranged for treatment with an analytic psychotherapist, who quickly recommended a boarding school. Once there, Wendy beat up the smaller children at the slightest provocation. Any form of reprimand from her teachers further flamed her rage.

After a year in the school, Wendy pleaded successfully to return to live with her newly remarried father. Father had undergone alcohol detoxification and rehabilitation and was now sober. Within weeks of her return, Wendy decided she hated her stepfamily and hit her stepsisters at every opportunity. This time father arranged for placement in a home for emotionally disturbed children, which ultimately led to her first hospitalization.

COURSE IN TREATMENT AT CHESTNUT LODGE

On admission to Chestnut Lodge, Wendy stated, "I have a habit of doing 'self-inflictions,'" and revealed scars from cuts on her arms and the inside of her legs. Wendy's paranoia was evident as she asked if there were tape recorders in the room. Her mood shifted rapidly from teenage ebullience to paranoid mistrust to anxious depression and agitation. Wendy asked for help with the following problems: her self-hatred and conviction that everybody else hated her, her mistrust of people, and her impulsivity. Wendy emphasized that she always remembered when people broke their promises. She complained of "hypochondriac tendencies"—for example, if she read about cancer then she believed she had the illness, and when she saw someone choking on food, she refused to eat for 3 days.

Her initial diagnosis at Chestnut Lodge was emotionally unstable personality, the DSM-II precursor to BPD. On the Wechsler Adult Intelligence Scale, administered at the time of her admission to the Lodge, Wendy's performance was within the average range, with a Full Scale IQ of 106. However, there was considerable intertest scatter attributed at the time to her limited education.

Wendy began treatment at Chestnut Lodge with Dr. Clair, a female psychiatrist, four times a week. In the first week, Wendy spoke straightforwardly about her difficulties and expressed "delight" over being at Chestnut Lodge because of the greater freedom afforded her. Staff who did not know her history thought she had no problems and presented as "friendly and adorable to everyone."

However, within 6 weeks of the admission, Wendy's deep distrust of human relationships revealed itself, as did her capacity for violence. She reported fantasies and dreams of people being dismembered. Wendy, now disappointed in Dr. Clair for unclear reasons, did not show for an appointment. That evening she tore Dr. Clair's nameplate from her office door, scratched the door, broke the ashtrays in the waiting room, and scattered the broken glass. Dr. Clair, frightened for her own safety, conducted the psychotherapy on the ward for the next 5 months.

Wendy began cutting herself regularly, at first secretly. She refused to acknowledge this behavior and reacted with extreme anger when anyone attempted to discuss it. To avoid her wrath, staff veered away from confrontation. The first time Dr. Clair learned of Wendy's cutting, she attributed it to Wendy's fear of an impending visit to a friend's home and so curtailed her privileges. However, it gradually became clear that Wendy developed a pattern of cutting herself every night while Dr. Clair was on night duty so that Dr. Clair would have to care for her. One evening, while once again suturing Wendy's bleeding arm, Dr. Clair confronted Wendy with this interpretation. Wendy felt Dr. Clair was being critical and responded with such intense agitation and anger that three aides were required to subdue her. Once quiet and released, Wendy pounced on Dr. Clair, ripping her blouse and scratching her face.

Wendy's self-mutilating behavior became a focus of staff concern and interest. Dr. Clair noted that Wendy cut herself when high as a way to calm down, when depressed as a way to feel better, and when she felt too "full" as a way to get rid of the people from the past who were crowding inside her. One staff nurse commented that Wendy cut herself at the slightest frustration. Another observed that Wendy always managed to be where a staff person could see her dripping blood. After each cutting episode, there appeared to be a release of tension and a period of giddiness and "kittenish" behavior.

Wendy spoke often of a feeling of depersonalization prior to cutting that she characterized as feeling dead and unable to feel her skin. During these states, Wendy was a detached observer and did not experience pain. Staff remarked that Wendy often had no real awareness that she had cut herself, but rather acted as though it were happening to someone else.

Dr. Clair observed that Wendy was reenacting her relationship with her parents within the therapeutic relationship. Wendy played both parent and child: fighting, ordering, accusing, and then wanting to be looked after or punished. In one session, Wendy, the beneficent parent, expressed a desire to teach Dr. Clair, who was from a foreign country, how to drive, improve her grammar, and learn American customs. During the next session, Wendy, now the child, brought clothes and asked Dr. Clair's advice on how best to wear them. Within moments, Wendy the punishing parent, declared a wish to whip Dr. Clair by tying her to a bed and beating her with belts. Next, the corrective parent, Wendy slapped herself on the face, called herself a nasty brat, and said, "Why do you do these things?"

The week of her eighteenth birthday staff held a special party for Wendy as family members had forgotten her. Her room was gaily decorated and full of presents. Briefly buoyed by this show of affection and concern, Wendy remarked that "maybe people like me for myself." However, within the week, she became depressed and depersonalized and walked around as though in a "fugue state," complaining that she had not accomplished anything in her life. She refused to eat, stating she felt "too full," and had to be tube-fed. She pleaded to be held, petted, and caressed, in great contrast to her prior refusals to be touched. Wendy clutched Dr. Clair's hands and asked to stroke her hair.

As Wendy recovered from this episode, Dr. Clair informed her that she was pregnant and leaving Chestnut Lodge in 1 month. Dr. Clair wrote that "a month of depression followed for both of us." Wendy alternated between expressions of bitter hatred of babies and cheerful protestations of happiness for Dr. Clair.

Their last meeting was held in Wendy's room. As Dr. Clair arrived, Wendy was spraying perfume. In a magnanimous farewell gesture, Wendy had arranged caviar, hearts of artichoke, coffee, and candy for Dr. Clair. She would not permit Dr. Clair to smoke her own cigarettes but offered hers from a silver case. Wendy apologized for her behavior and asked questions about Dr. Clair's pregnancy. As they said goodbye, Wendy conveyed intense sadness and fought back tears. Alone, Wendy walked to the nurse's station and asked an aide to comfort her. As he was busy, Wendy returned to her room and cut herself.

Dr. Mullen, who had come from Ireland for advanced training at Chestnut Lodge, was assigned to treat Wendy over the next 1½ years. He recalled her on his first day at the hospital as he carried bags to his new office on a snowy afternoon. Wendy stared at him as though he had "fallen from outer space." Dr. Mullen observed:

> She treats you like you were a magnet and surrounded by a very powerful magnetic field into which she is afraid to come, as though she herself is also somewhat of a magnet[,] and when these two fields conflict she gets disturbed. In a way I have also noticed that she moves around you, around this field[,] and suddenly stops transfixed, in a null point where the fields or lines opposed do not clash. She will look at you with feelings that are completely mixed. She can look at you with awe and great admiration and at the same time with complete disgust and fear. There is an emotional closeness and tremendous gap at the same time. I have felt that the therapy is finding these null points in which she can be comfortable and she can observe you and where you can be comfort-

able too because her magnetic field is also extremely intense. . . . It seems like you also have to condition yourself comfortably in order to be an observer of what is going on. In a way it has been like a dance where you are close enough to keep the rhythm but far enough not to be so intimate.

During the initial sessions, Wendy sat on the edge of Dr. Mullen's couch without making eye contact. She paced constantly and frequently left the office for a glass of water. Wendy chain-smoked, and when she was especially anxious, her leg vibrated. Wendy informed Dr. Mullen that she had chosen him because he was a man, a judge, and would not tolerate her destructive behaviors. She brought in a jumble of twisted wires that she said represented an empty chair and a woman with a baby in her arms who was Dr. Clair. Dr. Mullen thought it aptly portrayed Wendy's view of herself as "tangled, misshapen and unidentifiable."

Dr. Mullen learned to be careful not to express too much concern for Wendy or to act too human. When he did, Wendy sneered, "You stay on your side of the street, buddy, and I'll stay on mine." When upset with him, Wendy accused Dr. Mullen of being "high and mighty." On a day when Dr. Mullen was particularly worn down with administrative problems, Wendy informed him that all of the patients were complaining of their care. Dr. Mullen confided that he was having a rough day, and Wendy retorted, "Sob, sob . . . want me to shed a tear for you?" Dr. Mullen, now provoked said, "I dare you to." Wendy, feeling attacked, rebutted with, "I'd rather put a knife in your back."

Wendy had difficulty distinguishing Dr. Mullen from her father. She felt he accused her of cutting herself to get attention just as her father used to do when she had an accident or was ill. Wendy had frequent associations to older men being sexually interested in her. During one session, Wendy jumped in alarm on seeing Dr. Mullen's black raincoat behind the door, imagining him about to rape her. Early in the treatment Wendy came to one session wearing tight clothes and acting "giggly and seductive." She confessed, "I've done something terrible" and eventually confided to Dr. Mullen that she had slipped into a town bar the previous evening and accompanied a drunken man to his apartment. Feeling attracted to the handsome Dr. Mullen, Wendy accused the head nurse of recruiting student nurses to parade in front of Dr. Mullen so he could decide which one to date. During another session, Wendy confessed with, great embarrassment, her sexual excitement while petting her animals. She wished that she could feel as sexual with men. This confession was followed by wondering if Dr. Mullen was a "sex fiend."

Wendy frequently began sessions with statements such as "He's in a bad mood," "He's got a headache," "He has a hangover," and "He's depressed." Dr. Mullen understood that Wendy had learned to predict the mood of her parents before approaching them as a means of self-protection. After a trip to Chicago, Dr. Mullen returned with a small ivory elephant as a gift for Wendy. Although Wendy had talked with pleasure of receiving Dr. Clair's gifts, she stormed out of Dr. Mullen's office, shouting, "You actually mean it that you are going to give it to me?" Dr. Mullen followed Wendy to the ward and found her sitting in a fellow patient's room. Her anger was palpable, and despite Dr. Mullen's fear, he stayed his ground and questioned why Wendy had walked out in anger. She sat silently until Dr. Mullen glanced away. Within moments Wendy attacked him from behind, smashed two lamps on his head, and clawed and bit him. They wrestled for a speechless 8 minutes until an aide arrived and helped to subdue her. Once calm, Dr. Mullen again attempted to speak with her. Within seconds, Wendy again jumped on him and punched him. She was placed in a cold, wet sheet pack to calm down. Dr. Mullen acknowledged that he had no idea what Wendy was upset about.

Dr. Mullen sought consultation from his supervisor and was advised that he could not take care of Wendy's needs unless he took care of his own. Dr. Mullen then ordered that Wendy be placed in a sheet pack during their sessions. Now contained and apparently feeling safer, Wendy eventually was able to explain that she reacted violently because Dr. Mullen reminded her of her father. She said, "The only thing missing was you didn't reek from alcohol." At that moment, Wendy had apparently been unable to distinguish Dr. Mullen from her father. Dr. Mullen explained to Wendy that she had "misidentified" him and that he did not want to get beaten up because of this. He encouraged Wendy to work with him to recognize when she misidentified so that she could "hold the impulse a moment."

One session that Dr. Mullen recalled vividly during this time details the cumulative trauma of Wendy's young life. Wendy requested an emergency session because the head nurse, whom she liked, was leaving. Wendy cried bitterly during the following monologue:

> Everybody leaves me . . . my mother, my father . . . what little he was, he left me, too . . . my relatives, where are they? . . . as if I had dropped from the skies . . . no one ever calls or writes . . . how much I have longed to have parents and a home, but where? . . . what was I to do? . . . they let her die . . . she was weak and helpless, drinking, lonely and miserable . . . she was sick, hallucinating and paranoid, and the old man . . . I hate him . . . he beat her and nobody could do anything . . . what could I do? . . .

oh, you don't know Dr. Mullen, it's unbelievable . . . I can't understand how I lived through all this . . .

Wendy recalled her dogs, saying,

[T]hey would like it here . . . I could have died . . . they didn't want me . . . my father, he kicked me and hurt me, he banged my head on the ground, he kicked me in certain places [the genitals] . . . he didn't want to have a female child . . . once he attacked me when I returned from the club . . . he hit me on the ears and he knew how sore my ears were . . . I couldn't run . . . He told me he was going to take me out and kill me and I was so afraid . . . I shouted to Bessie to help me but she couldn't help me . . . that's a strange place, Dr. Mullen . . . you will never know . . . then he hit me and I ran and locked myself in the bathroom . . . I used to run to the barn and speak to the horse and tell the horse "please take me away" . . . then I would talk to the dogs.

Dr. Mullen's case presentation was fraught with misgivings and countertransference responses. Before summarizing the treatment, he informed staff that while on the phone with a patient on Wendy's ward, he heard Wendy in the background "raving like a maniac." Dr. Mullen expressed discouragement, as he had believed Wendy had improved. Her screams were like "a ghost coming back to haunt him."

Dr. Mullen admitted he was frightened during sessions that Wendy at any minute would spring at him with murderous rage. Wendy's "great seductiveness" to others made him feel jealous. Her manipulations coerced him into expressing his feelings. Dr. Mullen's recurring image was of them being on opposite sides of the street. Wendy hurled stones at him and hit the cars occasionally while he, dodging the stones, shouted across the din of the traffic. He stated, "I have to deal with my own feelings of self-preservation, hopelessness, rage and murder while trying to hurl interpretations at her. . . . It's not been easy."

Staff commented on how difficult it was to help Wendy. They were perplexed by her identity diffusion as she became manic like one patient, became catatonic like another, and cursed like a third. Another enduring feature of Wendy's condition was a preoccupation with physical illness. The list of Wendy's appointments with medical specialists in 1 month's time was staggering. She also was episodically anorexic. So poor was her behavioral regulation that it took six men to restrain her when angry and agitated. Thorazine and Cogentin, which were now prescribed regularly, did not prevent these outbursts.

At this point in the treatment, the hospital received a letter from Wendy's guardian stating that because of a recent stock market setback Wendy could no longer afford inpatient care and would have to become an outpatient within a month. Wendy expressed great fear over what would happen if she was to become violent outside of the hospital and there was no one to "put me down or beat me up and put me back."

Because of Wendy's financial situation, the focus shifted to moving her into the community. Wendy attempted work but was unable to keep a regular schedule and complained that the work was beneath her. Staff rented Wendy an apartment near the hospital and helped her furnish it. After moving, she became increasingly depressed with continuous suicidal ruminations. Without the structure of the hospital, she forgot to take her medications and became increasingly disorganized. She was readmitted as an inpatient but discharged 2 weeks later. After the police found Wendy wandering the streets several times in a confused state, they returned her to the hospital.

Pressure to move out of the hospital continued. Wendy made repeated efforts to contact relatives to take her home with them. No one responded. Staff observed increased fragmentation and loss of identity, and Wendy abandoned her request for discharge and initiated a transfer to a different hospital. Wendy reasoned that she needed a fresh start in a new place.

Wendy was transferred as scheduled to the new hospital and remained there until her twenty-first birthday 3 months later. She eloped 2 weeks later, and the hospital discharged her against medical advice.

FOLLOW-UP FIFTEEN YEARS LATER

The follow-up interview occurred 15 years after Wendy's discharge. At the time of the interview, not surprisingly, Wendy resided in a state psychiatric hospital. A recent hip surgery required intensive medical and psychiatric management, and Wendy was transferred from the board-and-care home where she had been living to the hospital. Wendy was maintained on 600 mg of Thorazine a day and was receiving supportive therapy one to three times a week as part of a research protocol.

The interviewer felt Wendy was psychotic because of her marked loosening of associations and irrelevant responses to some questions. She was also unable to provide a coherent chronology of her life.

Wendy had become a chronic patient—in the revolving door of hospitals, halfway houses, and downtown hotel rooms in four states. Wendy had married twice. Both husbands had been fellow patients whom she had met during hospital stays. Although still married to her second husband, Wendy was not cognizant of his location. Wendy, supported by a combination of money from her now-meager trust fund and from her father, with whom she had reconciled, lived below the poverty level. Wendy's social life centered around her mental health care providers and other patients. Carrie, her sister, visited about once a month, and Wendy visited father occasionally.

When asked what she regarded as her major psychiatric symptom, Wendy answered, "Anxiety," but added that rather than trouble her it made her "energetic." The interviewer learned that Wendy had demonstrated a pattern of Thorazine overdoses that had precipitated numerous brief hospitalizations. This behavior pattern resulted in a reputation as persona non grata in many halfway houses. Wendy acknowledged that she overdosed to obtain attention, even though she maintained it was not effective.

Wendy recalled Chestnut Lodge with nostalgia as an extremely pleasant and satisfying place. Work with Dr. Clair had been her best therapeutic experience. Although inarticulate about other questions, Wendy stated clearly that Dr. Clair had been a special person: "I liked everything about her . . . and felt very close to her." Wendy's major complaint was of "not liking to be restrained or in seclusion." She contrasted Chestnut Lodge positively to the many other hospitals to which she had been admitted.

Wendy's understanding of her illness was minimal, as evidenced by her statement that her diagnosis was passive-aggressive personality, which she thought meant that she had a passive and an aggressive personality. She then asked the interviewer if that was the same as being a schizophrenic.

Several weeks after the interview, Wendy phoned the director's office and requested a job in psychiatry. The call was transferred to the follow-up interviewer, who learned that Wendy had left the state hospital and moved into a downtown hotel. Wendy reiterated her desire to work and her interest in medicine, psychiatric nursing, and animals, and expressed confusion as to how to go about getting a job in these fields. Wendy seemed satisfied with encouragement to discuss her desires with her case manager and hung up after this brief exchange.

Some years later, Wendy was discovered in an educational film about community aftercare for the mentally ill. Wendy, now in a board-and-care home in the community, had become a mental health consumer spokesperson. In strident voice, Wendy complained of the inadequate care in the community and recalled fondly her days in Chestnut Lodge, her model for good care.

DISCUSSION OF ETIOLOGY AND OUTCOME OF DISORDER

Wendy's disorder was one of the most severe, and her outcome one of the worst, of the Chestnut Lodge BPD sample. Her case illustrates the most severe genetic and biological vulnerability with the most extreme forms of child maltreatment and adverse life events.

Etiology

Biological and Environmental Risk Factors

Wendy's case illustrates the developmental outcome of moderate to severe biological vulnerability interacting with severe maltreatment and cumulative trauma. Both parents were alcoholic and suffered from severe Cluster B personality disorders. Mother may also have suffered from psychotic depressions, and father reportedly evidenced "unusual thinking." Both of Wendy's brothers had alcoholism and severe personality dysfunction, one with antisocial personality disorder and the other, who had also been hospitalized at Chestnut Lodge, with BPD. The latter brother also suffered from severe depression and committed suicide.

Wendy suffered severe child maltreatment that included physical abuse, biparental neglect, emotional abuse, failure to protect, and possible sexual abuse by father's friends and possibly father. During the first 3 years of her life, both parents were physically absent; her father was overseas, and her mother was locked in her room. Wendy not only experienced abuse but witnessed physical violence between her parents on a regular basis. She witnessed other forms of parental dyscontrol, including promiscuity and verbal fights. Mother's early death further disorganized the family.

Her chaotic home life and her father's violence prohibited other children from playing with Wendy and compounded her isolation. She was unable to develop normal peer relationships, and her only form of play was with her troubled, possibly more disturbed, younger brother. Friends who visited the family also appeared to be alcoholic and disinhibited. Even the family live-in housekeeper, who fulfilled some parental functions, was alcoholic and neglected Wendy's need for protection by taking her to bars.

Protective Factors

It is difficult to find protective features in Wendy's life except for the family's wealth. It did enable her to obtain a protected living environment and treatment until it diminished when she was in her early 20s. Wendy reportedly was appealing as a young girl, as staff referred to her as "friendly and adorable." She had the extroverted style of many BPD patients when stable and was engaging. Each of her therapists at Chestnut Lodge liked and persisted with her despite the enormous strain and anxiety of the work. Later in her life, her father's ability to abstain from alcohol, remarry, and develop greater stability also provided some protection in the form of ongoing support. Similarly, her sister's greater ability to function and lend support helped. Finally, unlike Sylvia (see Chapter 5), Wendy did not abuse drugs or alcohol.

Outcome

Wendy continued to demonstrate a disorganized attachment pattern with an inability to sustain relationships or live outside of a protected environment, persistent dysregulation of emotion and behavior, and severe cognitive disorganization and poor reality testing. At her most stable, she exhibited a detached attachment mode as long as she was in a highly structure protected environment.

Cognitive Dysfunction

Paranoid ideation. Paranoia was a constant feature of Wendy's cognition. She assumed others were going to hurt or take advantage of her. This belief made Wendy hypervigilant and directed much of her behavior. At Chestnut Lodge, her violent outbursts were triggered by paranoid interpretations of her therapist's actions. Paranoia was also evident in Wendy's accusations to the staff of heterosexual and homosexual affairs.

Transient psychotic states. Wendy's disorder represents the psychotic end of the borderline spectrum. During her long years of treatment, there were numerous references to psychotic phenomena. Her violent assaults appeared prompted by paranoid states. She reported persistent "voices" of three people inside her head that were "causing confusion." These appeared to be related to extreme dissociation and cognitive disorganization. Her description of two of the voices as being similar to of those her mother and father and the third being that of an angel who sided with her therapist does not sound typical of hallucinations but, rather, may represent a stress response producing unintegrated fragmentary cognitions about her relationship with her parents. Wendy was tormented by these "people," as indicated by her statement that "the only way to silence them was to shoot her or give her a lobotomy."

Wendy's ideas about how to get rid of the voices further revealed her primitive thinking. She bruised her leg so that the vibrations would hurt the "people" inside. Her cutting, at times, was directed toward bleeding these people out. During one acute decompensation, Wendy ate cloth and stones.

Wendy also exhibited magical thinking in that she believed that she could cause other people's death through physical proximity. When she read about cancer, she believed that she had the illness. When Wendy saw a patient choking on food, she refused to eat for 3 days, fearing she would choke. Wendy's rationales for cutting herself also evidenced peculiar logic. She was "cutting her doctors down to size" or getting rid of the people from the past who were making her "full."

At termination from the hospital, it was noted that Wendy had not had psychotic episodes in 2 years. However, at follow-up Wendy's thinking was disorganized and odd and lacked good reality sense. The interviewer noted loosening of associations and irrelevant responses to questions.

Dissociation. Wendy often had feelings of depersonalization that she characterized as feeling dead and unable to feel her skin. Her frequent cutting appeared to break the depersonalized state. Wendy dissociated often and made frequent and dramatic shifts in her state of mind and attachment model. One moment she was violent and vengeful; the next, a cigar-smoking, swaggering boy; and yet another, a seductive and giggly girl. Her therapists were kept off balance by these shifts and unable to form a relationship with a core aspect of Wendy's personality. It was not possible to fully evaluate the presence of dissociation at follow-up, but we speculate that it persisted as evidenced by her continued cognitive disorganization.

Emotional Regulation

Affective instability. Throughout the follow-up, Wendy exhibited extreme mood lability and chronic dysphoria. Anxiety and irritability predominated despite treatment. Wendy did exhibit a modest improvement in her capacity to contain affect, most likely related to medication compliance, which enabled her to live in the community for periods of time. However, she appeared easily overcome by affect, as evidenced by her frequent overdoses.

Intense anger or lack of control of anger. The devastating consequences of multiple forms of child abuse on emotional development are typified by Wendy's case. Wendy experienced overwhelming anger and demonstrated complete dyscontrol in its expression. Frightening and danger-ous in its intensity, her rage knew no boundaries. The 3-year-old Wendy who ran through her home screaming and breaking things became the 16-year-old who attempted to choke her therapist and the 18-year-old who required six aides to subdue her. Fueled by her father's taunts and beatings, Wendy's fantasy life was filled with violent imagery of retribu-tion. Having been treated cruelly, she expected and anticipated cruelty from others. Wishes to knife her father and blind him with a bullwhip merged into violent actions against her therapists. As her father had de-meaned her, so Wendy demeaned and devalued others. As her father had terrorized her, so Wendy provoked fear and horror in others.

Wendy's violent outbursts during treatment were directed toward caregivers. There were no reports of assaults on other patients or strang-ers. These assaults appeared to be triggered by paranoid feelings of betrayal, threat, and violation. At these times, Wendy lost reality contact and was transformed into a wild animal fighting for survival. Often she seemed to relive an interaction with her father. If Wendy had a variant of a multiple personality disorder, she may have become one of the "people" she described inside her and acted accordingly.

The absence of an arrest record and Wendy's ability to live in the community for prolonged periods of time during the follow-up period suggested that she no longer resorted to physical violence. This is a re-markable achievement relative to her hospital behavior. We speculate that Wendy's ability to live in the community was related to the cumu-lative action of treatment, both psychotherapeutic and psychopharma-cological, and the absence of an intensive psychotherapeutic or other close relationship such as that provided at Chestnut Lodge. Wendy's role as consumer spokesperson for the mentally ill indicated that although anger continued to motivate her behavior, she had discovered a socially acceptable and constructive forum for its expression.

Behavioral Regulation

Impulsive/compulsive use of pleasurable behaviors. Because Wendy was in the protective milieu of hospitals throughout most of her adolescence, the full potential for impulsivity in these areas cannot be assessed. There were two reports that described Wendy leaving the hospital grounds without permission, getting drunk, and being sexually in-volved with men from the town. One of these liaisons resulted in an abortion. However, overall during her hospitalization, there appeared to be minimal drug abuse and promiscuous behavior. Wendy was frightened and repulsed by sexual contact, which, given her history, was not surprising. Her impulsivity expressed itself through cutting and assaultive behavior. Her disorganization was so extreme she could not maintain compulsive behavior.

At follow-up, Wendy's frequent Thorazine overdoses and repeated address changes suggested continued impulsivity. However, it is surprising that substance abuse did not appear to be a major factor in Wendy's course, since both her parents and brothers suffered from severe alcoholism. Wendy's overdoses seemed to be an impulsive response to a stressor and a manifestation of neither abuse nor addiction. Although the records lacked details about Wendy's marriages, the fact that she married former patients and had no idea of their whereabouts suggested impulsivity in this area.

Suicidal/self-mutilative.   Wendy did not attempt or threaten suicide throughout treatment. However, her cutting typifies the self-mutilating behavior of the borderline patient. By age 10 she was cutting herself, which she referred to as "self-inflictions," when hurt or angry. During parts of her treatment, she cut her arms daily. This behavior served multiple functions. It was a communication about her tortured emotional life and a means to engage others. Wendy's behavior illustrates the impulsive use of cutting as a behavioral coping mechanism and form of communication. It calmed her when anxious and lifted her spirits when depressed; it also brought her back to reality when depersonalized. Wendy endowed the cutting with magical powers, believing that it could get rid of the people inside of her and "cut [her] doctors down to size." Her behavior is illustrative of the ubiquitous nature of cutting for some borderline patients and also of the primitive and concrete thinking that underlies it.

Considerable attention was given to Wendy's cutting behavior early in her treatment. It was difficult to determine whether it decreased considerably over time or whether staff and therapists habituated to it. One therapist commented that Wendy eventually replaced cutting with less harmful bruising of herself. During her last days at Chestnut Lodge and following an upsetting family meeting, Wendy cut her thigh, stating that seeing her blood was a means to verify her existence, indicating that she still resorted to this behavior under duress. There was no mention of this behavior at follow-up. Instead, Wendy overdosed frequently, suggesting that self-destructive behavior continued to play a central role in the maintenance of her equilibrium. The records indicated that Wendy had persistent medical problems related to early physical abuse and frequent accidents. Perhaps her chronic pain and repeated medical procedures replaced her cutting behaviors.

Abandonment fears. Much of Wendy's behavior appeared organized around staving off feelings of abandonment. She was truly abandoned by her mother and father and was left very much alone during her hospital stays. As Wendy told Dr. Mullen, "Everybody leaves me . . . as if I had dropped from the skies. . . . how much I have longed to have parents and a home . . . " The absence of parental care made her feel invisible. To her first therapist, Dr. Palmer, she wrote movingly, "You don't have to say or do much but just fill my emptiness in a way that I know you are still there and that you are aware of me." After her last session with Dr. Clair, Wendy cut herself. Dr. Mullen speculated that the "people" Wendy described in her head were her protection against utter loneliness. As Dr. Mullen terminated his relationship with Wendy, she provided a moving description of the absence of a sense of self and evocative memory of a loving relationship: "I am just talking to myself; I'm just a cloud and you're a haze."

Unstable Intense Relationships

Wendy's interpersonal behavior exemplifies the extreme end of the borderline spectrum and persistent and severe disorganization of her attachment mode and consequent severe cognitive dysfunction and emotional and behavioral dysregulation. In her interaction with therapists, she displayed an extreme form of idealization and devaluation. Wendy swung between slavish devotion and violent reprisals. The requirement that Wendy be in sheet pack during many of her therapy sessions underlines the enormous effort it required for her to sustain a relationship. Her great need and hopefulness were so easily and bitterly disappointed. She pleaded with Dr. Palmer to continue talking with her and attributed his interest as her reason for living. Wendy treated Dr. Clair like a queen, showering her with gifts and attention followed by bizarre and frightening retaliation. Dr. Mullen captured the instability of her relatedness when he noted that Wendy could look at him with great admiration and awe followed by complete disgust and fear. Similarly, he noted that she could make him feel special or like the "lowest form of protozoa."

Aside from therapists and hospital aides, Wendy seemed unable to maintain any relationship. Only one friend was mentioned while Wendy was hospitalized in Chestnut Lodge, but the friendship ended with the girl running terror-stricken out of the hospital. Although boyfriends were noted, they were nameless. Unlike the relationships of the patients with better outcome, Wendy's lacked depth or sustained involvement. They did not serve as an interpersonal laboratory or transition to healthier functioning. Attempts to place her in foster homes were thwarted by her uncanny ability to set one family member against the other. Wendy seemed incapable of friendship and love. This pattern continued into the follow-up period.

The most striking feature of Wendy's interpersonal behavior was her violence. As a child, Wendy witnessed violence between her parents and was subject to her father's random cruelty when he was drunk. Her mother's meanness was bizarre and twisted. Although Wendy took solace in her animals, she witnessed and may have participated in her brother's perverse "play" behavior (i.e., choking and then reviving birds). All these experiences contributed to her assaultive behavior.

Identity Disturbance

Wendy's identity disturbance was profound. Her self-image was of a "congenital, hereditary, disturbed person." Wendy's development was so severely disrupted and traumatic that she was unable to achieve many developmental milestones. Her gender identity fluctuated, and at times, Wendy acted as a boy, smoking cigars and cutting her hair short. She was frightened of sexual relationships because she felt she was "one of the boys" and reported murderous impulses during sexual encounters. She did attempt to date, but she could feel close neither emotionally nor sexually. Her two marriages were impulsive and short-lived.

Wendy was unable to complete high school and never worked. She never developed independent living skills. At follow-up, she had assumed an identity as a career mentally ill patient. This identity did provide her a unique niche. The mental health community of hospitals, halfway houses, and board-and-care homes, along with fellow patients, doctors, and case managers, provided her with a role and function. Her work as a consumer spokesperson for the mentally ill was the one career for which she was sadly well prepared and in which she could be effective.

DISCUSSION OF TREATMENT

Comparison With Current Treatments

Unlike both Lillian and Susan, Wendy was treated with medications throughout her hospitalizations, and sheet packs were used to further contain her. Fortunately, today we have improved medications, and she would probably be prescribed a combination of an antipsychotic for her paranoia and transient psychotic states, a mood stabilizer to treat her lability and intense affect states, and an antidepressant during periods of depression. Even with these medications she would remain a challenging patient, but psychopharmacological treatment would enable her to take greater advantage of psychosocial interventions and to live more successfully in the community.

The adolescent Wendy would be in and out of residential care, with attempts at foster care in between. Much would depend on the sophistication of the mental health staff and quality of care. The optimal program would provide a behavioral modification approach to target her behavioral dysregulation and parasuicidal behaviors. We suspect that her care would be continuously disrupted because of the emphasis on community living and the resultant pressure to discharge prematurely. This might increase her frustration and anger and aggravate her tendency toward violence or might lead to greater suicide attempts. It is notable that although Wendy enacted frequent parasuicidal behaviors, there were no reports of attempted suicide while she was hospitalized at Chestnut Lodge—a fact that may be related to the stability she experienced in the hospital setting.

Today, Wendy would be able to continue her education through special programs for emotionally disturbed adolescents. Her only option at the time was to attend the local school, and her behavior was far too disruptive to be maintained in that setting. As a result, she never graduated from high school or received any vocational training.

As an adult, Wendy would today receive treatment that is similar to that described in the follow-up period. She would be assigned a case manager, receive maintenance treatment with medication, be hospitalized, and/or attend day treatment programs episodically and reside in a board-and-care or other supervised living situation. She might receive supportive individual therapy periodically and be engaged in a clubhouse model program for mentally ill patients. It is notable that Wendy was accepted into a research project, where she received up to three therapy visits a week. She must have retained some aspect of her engaging style that instilled the possibility of improvement through psychotherapy.

Therapeutic Factors

The asylum/village provided by Chestnut Lodge was the most beneficial aspect of Wendy's care. If ever anyone needed a stable living situation characterized by kindness, consistency, and good care, it was Wendy. Her case exemplifies the profound and tragic consequences of brutal childhood maltreatment and family disorganization coupled with severe underlying biological vulnerability. The severity of her disorder provides compelling support for the importance of long-term residential treatment for adolescents that incorporates behavioral modification and skills development according to a combination of psychosocial rehabilitation strategies and the Linehan model, which will be described in the last two chapters.

Both treating psychiatrists at Chestnut Lodge were consistent in their attempts to maintain a relationship with and understand Wendy despite extreme provocation and physical threat. This could be possible only within the safety of the residential setting. As we will elaborate further in the remaining chapters, the intensity of individual psychotherapy provided at Chestnut Lodge is contraindicated for BPD patients with Wendy's level of severity. However, the personal and professional qualities that Dr. Clair and Dr. Mullen exhibited are examples of what is required of those working with BPD patients. They were empathic, intellectually curious, kind, and nonreactive and used consultation well. Among these qualities, their nonpunitive stance was especially important. Also, although they attempted to use the technique of interpretation, which was then seen as a central to patient improvement, they were flexible and able to work in the "here and now," as exemplified by Dr. Mullen's trying to help Wendy to "hold the impulse" rather than enact it.

The fact that Wendy, over 15 years and after many other treatment experiences, recalled Dr. Clair and her experience at Chestnut Lodge as her best treatment is a powerful statement. We suspect that Wendy's 3 years at Chestnut Lodge during her late adolescence did make a difference between killing herself or someone else and being able to live, however tentatively, in the community.

Countertherapeutic Factors

The most deleterious aspect of the treatment was the intensive psychoanalytic psychotherapy and the expectation that she could benefit from it. The interpersonal and cognitive demand of such treatment triggered further disorganization of her coping abilities and prompted her psychotic states and violent behavior. The therapeutic relationship exposed her deep longing and need for a loving childhood while intensifying her disappointment that it could never be met. It was not possible to fully repair the damage done by the brutality and pervasive neglect of her childhood. The extreme form of child maltreatment she suffered in interaction with her biological vulnerability is akin to psychological quadraplegia. Nothing restores the ability to breathe unassisted and the ability to move about flexibly. Although it is important to instill hope and to work toward as much recovery as possible, one always requires extensive prostheses.

In addition to the frequency and intensity of the therapy, the use of traditional interpretation was particularly harmful to Wendy. Insight, the holy grail of many psychotherapies, is too often overvalued at the patient's expense, prompting exploration and interpretations that disorganize the already brittle patient. Interpretation requires a level of integration that Wendy neither had nor could achieve. She heard interpretations as a criticism and attack, which triggered feelings of victimization, paranoia, and rage. Similarly, too much kindness from Dr. Mullen, as when he brought back a gift from his trip, crossed the boundary into a perception of violent rape. Wendy could not distinguish a simple act of kindness from violent abuse.

The other countertherapeutic feature of the treatment was an overestimation of Wendy's psychological and real-life capacities. It is striking that when her insurance dwindled, staff felt she might be able to live independently in an apartment despite the fact that she had never demonstrated skill in self-care or lived alone. This, unfortunately, still happens today as adolescents who have lived in residential settings turn 18 and are expected to assume adult status. Also, the treatment program at Chestnut Lodge did not address development of skills in activities of daily living. This emphasis, which is now standard in day rehabilitation programs, was sorely lacking in Wendy's treatment.

Therapist Struggles

Wendy's case exemplifies the most challenging aspects of working with severely disordered BPD patients. Her interpersonal reactivity was so extreme that she switched rapidly from one simple attachment mode to the next and kept staff and therapists continuously off guard. She engendered a realistic fear of violence and concern for one's personal safety. Her quick temper, short of violence, frightened staff and interfered with setting needed limits. At the same time, staff overestimated her capacities because she could also be "friendly and adorable." Also, when Wendy described her childhood in moving and vivid detail, she conveyed greater capacity for "insight' than was actually present or possible.

Wendy was skillful at various forms of manipulation. Dr. Mullen admitted feeling jealous when she turned her favors on others. As evidenced by her loverlike behavior toward Dr. Clair, Wendy could lavish considerable charm and attention on those whom she wanted to keep close. These shifting states challenged her therapist's equanimity. Dr. Mullen's analogy of magnetic fields, in which one has to find the null points at which both parties can be comfortable, is apt. Similarly, his comment that his work with Wendy went best when they were "close enough to keep the rhythm but far enough not to be so intimate" underscores the importance of maintaining a close distance.

III

Treatment

Universal Features of Treatment

In this chapter and in Chapter 8 ("Recurrent Themes and Issues"), we cover the universal features of treatment with BPD patients based on the model elaborated in Chapter 1. Based on this model, the broad goals of treatment are to develop a more integrated and organized attachment system, foster emotional and behavioral regulation, elaborate cognitive structures, and establish a more cohesive sense of self or identity with improved self-esteem and greater self-agency. The more immediate goals are often to keep the patient alive, to minimize harm to self and community, and to improve quality of life. As the case histories illustrate, treatment progress is based on the severity of the disorder and the ability of the treatment team to sustain an affectionate, safe attachment and dialogue with the patient and to organize the form of asylum and village the patient's disorder requires.

EVALUATION

A complete and thorough clinical evaluation is essential for treatment planning. This evaluation includes collecting standard clinical data regarding the patient's chief complaint and current functioning, psychiatric history and treatment, comorbid conditions, mental status examination, medical problems, family psychiatric and treatment history, substance abuse history, and developmental, social, and family history. Once the clinician, from his or her assessment, judges that a patient meets the criteria for BPD, we recommend that special attention be focused on the following areas:

- Comorbid conditions
- Cognitive strengths and weaknesses
- Extent of dissociation
- Degree and type of child maltreatment
- Relationship history
- Preferred methods for emotional regulation
- Violence potential
- Physical health status
- Strengths (including abilities and talents) and resilience

Each of these areas needs special consideration for the purpose of treatment planning.

Comorbid Conditions

Comorbidity among BPD patients is the rule rather than the exception for several reasons. The underlying biological vulnerability of BPD patients predisposes them toward mood and anxiety disorders. Cognitive-processing problems predispose them toward cognitive disorganization and transient paranoid and psychotic states under stress. The crisis-prone lives of BPD patients place them under conditions of high stress, which exacerbates these underlying vulnerabilities. Overwhelming anxiety and dysphoria in the absence of adequate cognitive processing and affect regulation contribute to addictive behavior toward drugs and alcohol, sex, and food, which in turn generates additional disorders.

Consequently, it is not surprising that BPD is usually comorbid with a range of mood, anxiety, impulse, dissociative, substance abuse, and psychotic disorders (Tyrer et al. 1997). The greater the number and severity of comorbid conditions, the greater the degree of underlying biological vulnerability and developmental deviation and consequent functional impairment. At the severe end of the borderline spectrum, patients often meet lifetime prevalence criteria for multiple diagnostic groups. Although not the focus of this book, the degree of comorbidity prevalent in patients with BPD calls for a broader understanding of the interrelationships among Axis I disorders and the development of a dimensional system of classification.

Careful assessment of coexisting Axis I disorders is essential, because they represent considerable emotional suffering for the patient, dominate the clinical picture, and determine large amounts of the variance in treatment response, course, and outcome. Further, Axis I conditions dictate which medications will be used. Effective medication management reduces the overall suffering of the patient and enables her or him to make greater use of psychotherapeutic interventions. In many parts of the country, BPD patients are unable to obtain psychotherapeutic treatment because of inadequate or absent health insurance. The relationship formed with the psychiatrist and the medications prescribed will serve as the primary treatment.

Comorbidity with other personality disorders also occurs with great frequency (Fyer et al. 1988). The comorbidity among personality disorders, in addition to speaking to the need for a dimensional as well as a categorical approach to classification, has additional implications. As with Axis I disorders, the greater the number of Axis II disorders for which the patient meets criteria, the more severe the patient's dysfunction and impairment in living.

Even when the patient does not meet the full criteria for other personality disorders, she or he often exhibits personality traits that cross all three personality clusters (A, B, and C). This heterogeneity may point to temperament and trait factors and the multiple models of attachment and to the underlying immaturity and fluidity of the personality structure. The relative strength of each of these traits influences the style of relating and the variations in treatment course. For example, the patient with greater antisocial and paranoid features will have more difficulty engaging in treatment and will have a higher likelihood of violent behaviors. Obsessive and compulsive traits may contribute to greater success in school, work, and daily living or, at the extreme end, to greater impairment.

It is also important to assess patients for the presence of substance abuse disorders. There is a strong link between abuse of alcohol, opioids, and other substances and BPD (Brooner et al. 1993; Drake et al. 1994; Helzer and Pryzbeck 1988; Links et al. 1995). The prevalence for co-occurring BPD among substance abusers is reported to be 21% (Poling et al. 1999). BPD patients may go on episodic binges during periods of high stress or develop physical and/or psychological dependence. Their chronic misery, poor affect regulation, and great discomfort with being alone make the use of drugs and alcohol compelling. Substance abuse further disinhibits behavior and is one of the leading immediate precipitants of suicide attempts and violent behavior and successful suicides and homicides. Short of these most tragic consequences, continuous drug abuse and dependence contributes to mounting health and interpersonal problems and an escalating downward spiral in functioning. Three out of four of the patients whose cases are presented in Part II used substances as a means of affect regulation. The unfolding of Sylvia's life (see Chapter 5) exemplifies the most tragic course and underscores the importance of including a treatment plan for addressing substance abuse problems.

Cognitive Strengths and Weaknesses

To assess cognitive abilities, we recommend that a careful history be taken of neurological problems, learning disabilities, and school and work functioning. Although we recommend psychological testing as needed and described later in this chapter, there are often insufficient resources to conduct such an evaluation. Therefore, the clinical interview must be especially thorough in obtaining information about cognitive problems. The interview should explore early neurological and developmental problems, language delays, learning disabilities, attentional problems, and medical problems that can impact cognitive functioning, such as head injuries and seizure disorder. The patient should be asked about her or his performance and grade averages in grade school, high school, and college. Successful completion of high school or college does not rule out learning disabilities, attention-deficit/ hyperactivity disorder (ADHD), or other cognitive problems, and neither does successful work performance. The individual may have learned to compensate for cognitive problems in school and work yet remains vulnerable in new situations. Residual effects will continue to interfere with performance and learning. Cognitive problems are overshadowed by the intense affects and dramatic behaviors of BPD patients and often go undetected.

To assist in establishing the presence of cognitive problems, the following tests, which have been found to be sensitive to the borderline disorder, may be administered for screening purposes:

- Rey-Osterreith (Lezak 1983; Osterreith 1944)
- Ruff Figural Fluency (Ruff et al. 1987)
- Digit Symbol (Wechsler 1958, 1981)
- Corsi/Block Span (Milner 1971)
- Embedded Figures (Witkin et al. 1971)

- Road-Map Test of Direction Sense (Money 1976)
- Wechsler Memory Scale—Logical Memory Test (Wechsler 1945)

A measure of overall intellectual functioning is also helpful in treatment planning and as a further screen for other cognitive problems. Fuller neuropsychological assessment may be warranted to assist with vocational referral and training or to establish the presence of specific learning disabilities or adult attention-deficit disorder.

Dissociation

Dissociation, as a manifestation of cognitive processing problems, requires special attention. Evaluating the extent of dissociation and assigning it as a primary target for treatment are essential. The patient should be queried about how frequently they experience dissociative phenomena. These phenomena include 1) *amnesia,* which refers to loss of memory for aspects of personal history; 2) *absorption,* which refers to one's becoming so engrossed in an activity that one is completely unaware of surroundings; and 3) *depersonalization,* which refers to the feeling of being disconnected from one's body or feelings. One measure that can be used to assess dissociation and its components is the Dissociative Experiences Scale (Bernstein and Putnam 1986).

Dissociation can also be observed during the interview when the patient becomes silent and stares into space for relatively long periods of time. Also, dissociation is present when the patient exhibits a lapse in reasoning as she or he describes experiences of child maltreatment or significant loss or when affect intrudes unexpectedly in the narrative. An example of a common occurrence of dissociation is when a patient describes being beaten with a matter of fact emotional tone or describes the grim details of a suicide plan with detached demeanor.

We speculate that patients who exhibit frequent and pervasive dissociation are at greatest risk for harm to self and others. As suggested in Chapter 1 ("An Integrated Developmental Model"), more severe dissociation may point to greater underlying biological vulnerability and cognitive processing problems. It may also reflect a more disorganized attachment pattern and greater impairment in the ability to process and integrate emotional information into meaningful cognitive schemas.

Child Maltreatment

To assess child maltreatment, the clinician must inquire about the presence, type, and severity of emotional and physical neglect and sexual, physical, and emotional abuse. The therapist must be sensitive to the probability that patients who are new to treatment may never have talked about these experiences or thought of themselves as a maltreated child. The patient does not have a coherent organized memory of her or his relationship with parents and will provide information in disorganized fragments. Within the same paragraph, she or he may describe totally different childhood experiences without observing the contradiction (e.g., that the patient's childhood was good and that father beat her or him regularly). The early revelation of child maltreatment can trigger powerful emotions and, before the therapeutic alliance and holding environment are fully in place, disorganize the patient and prompt regressive behavior such as binge drinking or cutting behavior. As this information is elicited, the clinician should minimize exploration but convey both empathy and containment and indicate that these matters will be dealt with gradually.

The Childhood Trauma Questionnaire (Bernstein et al. 1994), an instrument that probes for emotional and physical neglect as well as physical and sexual abuse, can be helpful. The emotional distance permitted through filling out a questionnaire enables the patient to provide information on the presence, type, and extent of maltreatment that can be discussed gradually over the course of treatment, if at all. However, even the questionnaire may spark emotional distress that will need to be addressed.

Relationship History

Obtaining a detailed history of relationships will help the clinician assess the level of disorganization and instability in attachment and will suggest the degree to which a more organized attachment mode can be formed. Further, this information will guide the treatment plan and may suggest the course of the therapeutic relationship. Areas to probe include the quality and length of past and current relationships with family members, friends, romantic partners, supervisors, and co-workers. Also, the clinician should ask about the quality, course, and length of relationships with prior mental health professionals.

Preferred Methods for Emotional Regulation

Because the most predictable yet potentially destructive feature of BPD is the potential for harm to self and other, the patient's preferred methods for regulating high arousal states must be evaluated. This evaluation includes a detailed review of present and past compulsive behavior patterns and impulsive acts. Of special concern is the type, extent, and frequency of self-mutilation, suicidal rituals, sexual behavior, eating disorders, and substance abuse. As these areas are discussed, the therapist assesses the potential for harm and identifies and highlights emotional regulation as a central focus of treatment.

Violence Potential

Finally, because of the pervasive anger that BPD patients experience, the clinician should assess the patient's potential for violence toward others (Meloy 1987). In general, the best predictor of future violence is a past history of violent acts. With this in mind, the clinician must elicit the patient's history of aggressive and violent acts. Antisocial, paranoid, and narcissistic personality traits serve as predisposing factors for violent behavior. The patient's skill and comfort level with knives, guns, and other lethal weapons and their availability also raise the threshold for violence. Of equal importance is an assessment of the presence and extent of substance abuse, as this feature amplifies the potential for violence in those so prone.

Physical Health Status

BPD patients often develop a variety of health problems related to early maltreatment and poor self-care. Substance abuse, self-mutilation, suicide attempts, promiscuity, and eating disorders also contribute to health problems. These problems become chronic and more debilitating as the patient ages. Thus, it is important to elicit current and past medical problems during the evaluation and include attention to health and coordination with health providers as part of the treatment plan. BPD patients often underreport or overreport health problems or have difficulty with clear descriptions. Further, they bring their intense and unstable form of relatedness to the health care arena, which often interferes with adequate care. We discuss this issue further in the section on psychopharmacological treatment.

Strengths (Including Abilities and Talents) and Resilience

An equally importance aspect of the initial and ongoing evaluation is the identification of patient strengths and resilience. As the case histories in this book illustrate, these qualities and abilities serve as protective factors and form the basis for positive development. The ability to work is an importance source of self-esteem and daily structure. Hobbies and creative abilities are areas that patient and therapist can use to develop greater tolerance for being alone and bearing distress as well as to develop self-esteem and a stronger sense of self. Outcome studies (McGlashan 1986; Stone et al. 1987) have suggested that patients with high intelligence, special skills, and physical attractiveness have better outcomes. These qualities, as reflected in the lives of Lillian, Susan, and Sylvia, have high social valence and enable the patient to negotiate in the world. A psychosocial rehabilitative approach that focuses on enhancing education, work skills, abilities, and talents provides the long-term foundation for improved functioning.

TREATMENT GOALS

The general goals of treatment with BPD patients are as follows:

1. Prevent suicide and/or homicide
2. Develop emotional and behavioral regulation
3. Reduce or eliminate harmful addictive behaviors
4. Stabilize and integrate attachment patterns
5. Facilitate the development and maintenance of a stable, sustaining physical and psychological environment
6. Treat mood, anxiety, and psychotic disorders with appropriate medications
7. Preserve and build social and work functioning to the fullest extent possible

We hope that the integrated model and case histories presented in this book will provide mental health professionals with greater optimism that these goals can be reached within the patient's capacities. The most important caveat is that treatment must be tempered and guided by a realistic appraisal of the patient's developmental level, capacities, and resources and that progress must be measured within that framework.

IT TAKES A VILLAGE

An African shibboleth says, "It takes a village to raise a child." At whatever age BPD patients enter treatment, they are developmentally immature and in need of protection and care. The degree of disorganization and instability in their attachment patterns causes them to engage their whole community—family, friends, employers, colleagues, and health, social welfare, and mental health professionals—in unstable and intense interactions as they attempt to get their needs met. Consequently, the disorder extracts a high price from the individual and society. For these reasons, an integrated community response is essential for effective treatment. The complexity of the disorder and the degree of the patient's needs usually require a team approach. The behavior wrought by the disorder is often too anxiety provoking and difficult for one person to bear alone. Single parenting of a challenging child without family and community support is fraught with troubles, and so it is for the solitary therapist working with a BPD patient.

Asylum and Village

The unique aspect of treatment at Chestnut Lodge was the provision of asylum and a village of concerned and caring people. This "holding environment" (Winnicott 1965) replicated aspects of a "good enough" home environment. Housing, food, structure, routine, activities, rituals, and emotional support were provided. Patients were provided a safe place and a community within which they could develop to the best of their abilities—an experience they missed or that was sorely disrupted in childhood.

All of us are sustained by supportive daily contacts with family, friends, co-workers, neighbors, and salespeople. The BPD patient's fragmented interpersonal models and unintegrated experience interfere with developing a cohesive social environment. Our mental health care and social service systems must aspire to providing asylum and village. The treatment team and mental health community are the core of this village, but physical health care providers and social service providers also are important participants.

Treatment Team

The psychotherapy provided at Chestnut Lodge was the cornerstone of the treatment provided for BPD patients. The therapeutic relationship remains the cornerstone of treatment today. However, as at Chestnut Lodge, the establishment of a treatment team that combines the functions of therapist, psychiatrist, and case manager is necessary. Akin to how many parents divide parenting functions, the therapist provides steady support and facilitates a dialogue about the patient's experience and the therapeutic relationship. The psychiatrist provides psychopharmacological treatment but also serves as an additional form of support to the patient and offers another interpersonal learning experience.

The case manager provides assistance with establishing a life structure, including financial stability, housing, food, vocational assistance, and community connections, while also serving as a supportive person in the patient's life. As life crises arise around basic needs, the case manager is available to advocate for and provide assistance to the patient. Both psychiatrist and case manager must be able and willing to discuss problems within their relationship to the patient.

TREATMENT PLANNING AND RESOURCES

With BPD patients, as with all patients, treatment must be tailored to the particular problems, strengths, limitations, and resources of the patient. In general, the acuity and chronicity of symptoms and the degree of functional impairment and social disability will dictate treatment, as we saw in the case vignettes. The availability of health insurance and a coordinated public mental health service often determines the kind and quality of care the patient can receive. In addition to the guidelines described below, we recommend the American Psychiatric Association's *Practice Guideline for the Treatment of Patients With Borderline Personality Disorder* (American Psychiatric Association 2001) and John Gunderson's *Borderline Personality Disorder: A Clinical Guide* (Gunderson 2001).

Severity of Disorder

Severe Impairment

Patients at the severe end of the borderline spectrum require a prosthetic approach to treatment that provides structure and life-long supportive mental health and social services (i.e., a continuous safe attachment). They also can benefit from a psychosocial rehabilitative approach that maximizes strengths and talents and fosters improved community functioning. These patients will have experienced the most severe forms of child maltreatment in the midst of the greatest biological vulnerabilities and exhibit the greatest impairment. The need for a prosthetic treatment approach for patients with severe impairment is illustrated by the cases of Sylvia and Wendy (see Chapters 5 and 6, respectively), who manifested high comorbidity, had chronic functional disability, relied on Social Security Disability insurance or family assistance, and required frequent hospitalizations and/or long-term residential care.

Moderate Impairment

At the moderate level of impairment, the patient will have moderate levels of either biological vulnerability or environmental risk factors with some protective factors. Their functioning, like Susan's (see Chapter 4), is characterized by fluctuating ability to work and maintain relationships and episodic disorganization. Treatment will usually involve psychotherapy and medication on either a continuous or an intermittent basis and intermittent hospitalization during suicidal crises or behavioral regressions. The patient may need periodic case management and social service assistance, depending on the presence of adverse life events and financial stability. These patients can also benefit from psychosocial rehabilitative strategies to develop or maintain work and role function.

Mild Impairment

Patients with the least dysfunction will usually exhibit milder biological vulnerability and greater environmental risk factors. They will require primarily psychotherapy and psychiatric treatment without use of case management and social welfare assistance. Hospitalization will be rare except during a major depression and suicidal crisis. As Lillian's case illustrates (see Chapter 3), patients with mild impairment are generally able to maintain work functioning, often at a high level, although breaks may occasionally occur. Work problems will revolve around conflicts with co-workers and bosses. General social functioning will be maintained, although it will fluctuate according to perceived mistreatment or availability of support. Intimate relationships will be the sources of greatest difficulty. Those closest to the patient may be aware of a certain intensity and fragility.

Public and Private Resources

Most BPD patients require long-term care, either ongoing or intermittent. Although there are no studies on the cost to society of untreated individuals, we estimate that the cost is high if costs for health care and social services, such as emergency room visits, medical treatment, child protective services, Supplemental Security Insurance (SSI), and the criminal justice system, are considered. Thus, we recommend that these general treatment features be applied creatively depending on the resources available to the patient.

Patients who have sufficient personal or family income and/or indemnity insurance to pay for private treatment will, depending on the community, be able to obtain ongoing treatment from a psychotherapist and a psychiatrist. Patients living in states that have passed mental health parity legislation should also have sufficient coverage to receive adequate care. However, insurance coverage usually must be based on a diagnosis of a DSM-IV Axis I condition and not BPD, which, at the time of writing, is not considered a covered diagnosis through the mental health parity legislation. Given the extent of comorbidity with Axis I disorders, this should not be a problem. However, the mental health community should also advocate that BPD, given the morbidity and mortality of the disorder, be included as a parity diagnosis.

In states that have not passed parity legislation, it may be advisable to convert insurance coverage for inpatient days to outpatient or day-treatment days to extend the availability of outpatient visits. If the maximum number of allowable visits per year is fewer than 20, the therapist might best serve the patient through education about the disorder, crisis intervention, and referral to a low-fee community therapist or therapist-in-training. The managed care psychiatrist would maintain the patient on medications and arrange hospitalization as needed. The therapist could serve as a case manager and be available as backup to the low-fee or training therapist in times of crisis.

Many HMO plans provide a minimum of 20 visits per year, not including medication management visits. Treatment can be organized so that the therapist can see the patient weekly for four to six sessions to build the alliance and then reduce visits over time. Some programs are making the investment to train staff in the dialectical behavior therapy (DBT) skills training approach developed by Marsha Linehan (1993a, 1993b). This treatment combines behavior therapy and skills training with traditional psychotherapeutic principles and mindfulness meditation. It offers both individual and group methodologies for work with the borderline client. Although the group treatment is designed to work in tandem with individual therapy, some organizations are experimenting with using the skills-based group modules in combination with an individual case management approach or on an individual coaching basis.

More severely disordered BPD patients and/or those without insurance are usually treated within public mental health systems that become the patient's asylum and village. Within these systems, an institutional alliance is forged. The standard of care in public mental health settings varies greatly depending on the area of the country, social policy, and available funding. The general standard in community mental health centers is the provision of a case manager and a psychiatrist. Some communities are now using an approach based on the Program of Assertive Community Treatment (PACT) model (Allness and Knoedler 1998), which relies on a team of case managers and community aides who are available to the patient 24 hours a day in the community to prevent or minimize continuous crises and hospitalizations. Psychosocial rehabilitation treatment models, which emphasize quality of life and maximizing the patient's ability to function in the community, are also becoming more widely available.

In some programs, mental health trainees provide services. Because training rotations are usually 1 year, the patient must adjust to these transitions. This adjustment is facilitated by the knowledge that the clinical supervisor usually remains constant, as do the clinical administrators who oversee the patient's care. It is helpful for the patient to meet the supervisor or administrator so that he or she is a real presence in the patient's life. As needed, the patient can call on the supervisor as one might an aunt, uncle, or grandparent for special assistance. Also providing continuity within the public mental health system are permanent business and custodial staff. These familiar and friendly faces are supportive to the patient and become part of their village.

In public mental health systems that are only able to provide crisis intervention, medication maintenance, and hospitalization, the relationship with the psychiatrist is central. However, we advocate that BPD patients be provided with an ongoing case manager/therapist within the public mental health center, because most psychiatrists have extremely high caseloads and do no have the time available for the BPD patient. The lack of availability of psychiatrists can increase social service, health care, and criminal justice costs.

Day Treatment and Hospitalization

For patients with minimal daily structure and high acuity demonstrated by frequent hospitalizations related to suicidal behaviors and self-mutilation, a partial day treatment program can provide needed structure and containment. These programs combine socialization activities with behavioral skills training and vocational assistance to help stabilize the patient. Involvement in these programs can last from 6 months to several years. After completing the program or on obtaining maximal benefit from this approach, the patient usually returns to an individual therapist/case manager and psychiatrist for ongoing maintenance.

The use of hospitalization for BPD patients is controversial, as some feel it encourages too much regression and, in a sense, rewards "bad" behavior (e.g., self-mutilation and suicide attempts). The brief duration of hospital stays now dictated in many parts of the country by tighter control on hospital costs makes it almost impossible to err in this direction. However, we believe that hospitalization in either a locked or open facility is a clinically necessary treatment option for BPD patients. The major function of hospitalization is containment; to help the patient feel securely attached to the treatment team, to reduce high arousal levels, and to prevent harmful behaviors. As the patient feels contained and secure with the treatment team and her or his living situation stabilizes, the need for hospitalization rapidly disappears.

The most obvious indications for hospitalization are when the patient is seriously suicidal and suffering from major depression or undergoing a transient psychotic episode with paranoia and disorganized behavior. For patients with fewer psychological and social resources and greater cognitive impairment, hospitalization is often needed to protect the patient and others from increasingly disorganized and self-destructive behavior. The goal of hospitalization is protection for the patient and her or his significant others, stabilization, assurance of medication compliance, reinforcement of coping skills, and reconnection to the outpatient treating team. Close communication among all care providers is essential so that the patient feels that the safety net extends back and forth between inpatient and outpatient services. Attempts at interpretation or discussing underlying causes usually are ineffective and often exacerbate distress. Instead, the patient requires the predictable routine of a hospital, where she or he experiences the environment as containing and structuring. This facilitates the reduction of unmanageable emotional states and behavioral dyscontrol.

Patients who are able to work generally do not want hospitalization. They rely on their work for structure and containment, and the workplace serves as their day treatment program during crises. Nonetheless, hospitalization may be necessary during suicidal crises. Such crises can occur in the midst of a major depression or significant life event and during any serious disruption in important relationships, including the therapeutic alliance. The potential lethality of higher-functioning patients should never be underestimated.

The enforced routines and hierarchical structure of an inpatient ward or short-term residential facility can bring out the worst in BPD patients as they reexperience being at the mercy of arbitrary authority. The range of personality styles of inpatient and residential staff challenges BPD patients' interpersonal repertoire and coping ability. As will be discussed in greater detail later, even during short stays, these patients quickly divide staff into those they perceive as the "good" (more flexible and caring) staff and those they perceive as the "bad" (more rigid, punitive, and blaming) staff and rely on the former while provoking the latter. This tendency to split staff speaks to the importance of staff training and the development of a coherent approach to working with BPD patients. The greater the staff cohesion, the more likely the patient will improve.

APPROACHES TO INDIVIDUAL, GROUP, AND FAMILY PSYCHOTHERAPY

There are currently two major approaches to the psychotherapeutic treatment of BPD patients: psychodynamic and cognitive-behavioral. Psychodynamic approaches are exemplified by the manualized transference focused psychotherapy (TFP) developed by Kernberg and his colleagues (Clarkin et al. 1999). This approach is based on a theoretical understanding of BPD in terms of object relations. TFP, like other psychodynamically based treatments, focuses on the emotionally laden themes that emerge in the here and now of the relationship and relies on techniques of clarification, confrontation, and interpretation within the transference relationship. Preliminary findings of an uncontrolled outcome study of manualized TFP found a decrease in suicide attempts, fewer hospitalizations, and fewer number of hospital days after 1 year of treatment (Clarkin et al. 2001).

Cognitive-behavioral approaches, as exemplified by the work of Marsha Linehan (1993a, 1993b, 1995), are based on cognitive-behavioral theory with an emphasis on behavioral learning theory. In her DBT approach to BPD patients, Linehan has added principles of dialectical thinking, validation strategies, and mindful meditation to the behavioral approach. Through the melding of these streams of thought, she has developed a comprehensive theory-based and stagewise approach to treatment that incorporates individual therapy, manualized group-based skills training (Linehan 1993b), clear guidelines for crisis availability, and integration of pharmacotherapy. Her approach emphasizes the importance of a regular team collaboration and consultation. She has conducted a number of treatment outcome studies (Linehan et al. 1993, 1994) that suggest that DBT results in a reduction in parasuicidal behavior, fewer inpatient hospital days, improved social functioning, and reduction in drug abuse. Her approach is receiving wide attention because of its efficacy. Also, its manualization enables clinicians to apply it in a wide variety of settings and lessens their feelings of helplessness and anxiety. The highly structured nature of the approach and its emphasis on close teamwork and collaboration also help to contain clinician anxiety and countertransference reactions that interfere with treatment.

Family therapy can be an important aspect of treatment when the family pays for treatment, the patient is still living at home, or the patient maintains significant involvement with the family. There is a general consensus that family therapy is most effective when a structured psychoeducational approach is used in either a single-family or a multiple-family group setting. Current approaches have evolved from work based on theories on the role of expressed emotion in the families of patients with schizophrenia or bipolar disorder and the importance of education and family support in the treatment of serious mental disorders. Two primary models are currently in use. One was developed at McLean Hospital and is now in manualized form (Berkowitz and Gunderson 2002). The other was developed at the Westchester Division of New York Hospital and employs DBT-based exercises (Hoffman 1999; Hoffman and Hooley 1998). The general strategy of these approaches is to educate the family about the borderline diagnosis and about how to create a calmer and more predictable home life.

In summary, the psychotherapeutic treatment commonly used today with BPD patients is a practical mix of psychodynamic (including psychoanalytic and self psychological–based methods), psychoeducation, cognitive-behavioral, and psychosocial rehabilitative approaches. Gunderson (2001) has written a comprehensive guide to the use of multiple treatment modalities based on treatment goals and expectable changes that integrates his many years of clinical and research experience with approaches of other major contributors in the field. In addition, he elucidates the generic therapeutic processes of containment, support, structure, involvement, and validation and the functions they serve as the core of any psychotherapeutic treatment with BPD patients.

Our discussion of treatment mirrors the work of Gunderson in that work with BPD patients must integrate all available modalities and employ the generic psychotherapeutic and educational processes he describes. Our discussion focuses on further elaboration of the generic principles of treatment on the basis of the etiological model and case histories.

THERAPIST QUALITIES

Work with BPD patients is not for everyone, although most mental health professionals will encounter borderline patients at some point in their career. Effective work requires certain qualities in the psychotherapist. Central to all therapies and critically important with borderline patients is *empathic capacity*. The therapist has to be able to look into the "heart of darkness" without being overwhelmed with anxiety, fear, disgust, or pity. Included in empathic capacity is the ability to gauge what the patient needs from the therapist in terms of limits, mirroring, affective regulation, and human connection. Flexibility and creativity within an ethical and commonsense frame of reference not only are essential but make the work challenging and rewarding. Patience is important, as BPD patients fluctuate markedly in their mood and behavior—one moment an insightful adult conversing articulately and the next, a primitive wild child communicating through knife cuts on the arm. Also, the work is slow, and the tortoise wins the race.

A capacity for introspection and a willingness to seek consultation as needed are two other key qualities. The therapist needs to immerse himself or herself in the inner world of the patient to intuit how to respond effectively. The chaotic and primitive inner states of the patient can be frightening, anxiety provoking, and depleting, and the therapist needs a strong collegial support system, his or her own "village," on which to rely. The collegial village serves to protect therapist and patient. The most common challenge for the therapist is how to maintain a distant closeness. Both therapist and patient are in danger of seduction and abuse. The therapist, novitiate or experienced, must accept his or her own need for support and consultation throughout the therapeutic process.

Another quality that helps sustain the therapy is curiosity about what motivates human behavior. BPD patients teach us much about the shadowy corners of the mind but also about human resilience in the face of staggering adversity. A detective-like curiosity helps us to understand the complex puzzle of borderline behavior and to help our patients see the adaptation and will to live in what appears as self-destructive and murderous behavior. A sense of humor and the use of humor strengthen the therapeutic bond and provide balance to the intensity of the therapy. Humility in the face of the tragic and heroic efforts of the patient to survive and maintain human connection provides perspective.

A SECURE BASE: THE THERAPEUTIC RELATIONSHIP

As Bowlby (1988) noted, the "continuing potential for change . . . means that at no time of life is a person invulnerable to every possible adversity and also that at no time of life is a person impermeable to favorable influence. It is this persisting potential for change that gives opportunity for effective therapy" (p. 136). The psychotherapeutic relationship is at the heart of the long-term treatment effort with the BPD patient. We suspect that it is rare that BPD patients develop a secure, organized attachment model with full empathy, interpersonal flexibility, and capacity for intimacy, even with the best treatment. However, treatment does provide the patient with a chance to develop a more stable and integrated attachment schema. The safe, supportive, caring, educative, containing, and structuring aspects of treatment experienced over time contribute to real interpersonal skill and knowledge. The multiple modes are gradually integrated, to the extent possible, through the action of new primary affective experiences with treatment team members. This development may take several forms, and it is these differences that contribute to the differences in outcome.

We have chosen the metaphor of the BPD patient as psychologically deaf and blind, a child bewildered by human relationships and without a language to voice her or his inner confusion. Akin to Annie Sullivan's work with Helen Keller (Keller 1903), the therapeutic relationship enables the patient to develop the use of language in order to give voice and narrative to her or his experience. In so doing, treatment helps the patient to see the world of human relationships more clearly, tame her or his wild heart, and become civilized and learn the ways of social discourse.

The model for this process is Bowlby's (1969/1982) concept of a goal-corrected partnership described in Chapter 1 ("An Integrated Developmental Model"). The treatment team establishes a dialogue with the patient about needs, wants, plans, and goals. Patient and team embark on a process of translating and decoding dense and convoluted action patterns or sensorimotor schemas into language and back into direct and more effective interpersonal action. What evolves is a model of a more cooperative and interdependent relationship.

As discussed earlier, the relational problems that BPD patients experience emanate from multiple contradictory states of mind regarding what to expect from others. They expect that they will be hurt, deprived, neglected, disappointed, abused, manipulated, or exploited and simultaneously hope that they will receive care that meets their specific needs within the context of unconditional love and respect. The behaviors of BPD patients correspond directly and indirectly to how they were treated and how they learned to cope with the real circumstances of their early environment. The clearer these links are to the therapist and, to the extent possible, the patient, the more understandable the patient's behavior becomes.

The wish for care and protection from neglect is inchoate, unlike the expectation of harm toward which the BPD patient has developed elaborate survival strategies. It is a wish and hope without articulation and definition. Its powerful presence is felt by the therapist through the pull he or she feels from the patient for special treatment and perfect attunement to the patient's needs. It is felt through the terrible disappointment the patient experiences when the therapist does not meet these magical expectations. The expectation of abuse, on the other hand, suffuses the wish for closeness with heightened wariness about potential attack. The beloved becomes the target of suspicion as well as yearning. These dichotomous sets of expectation or states of mind result in intense and unstable relatedness and the swings between idealization and devaluation that characterize BPD relationships.

The medium for change lies within the therapeutic relationship and community, where the patient experiences being understood and learns about reciprocity and about what one can get from others and what one must provide for oneself. Expectations of harm and deprivation never fully disappear but are gradually modified by the patient's actual experiences with the therapeutic community.

INITIATION OF TREATMENT

BPD patients may first enter treatment through a hotline, a SWAT team encounter, an inpatient stay, an emergency room visit, or a traditional outpatient appointment. Whatever the point of entry, the initial contact with a BPD patient is often memorable by its intensity. The therapist feels swept into the patient's emotional vortex and struggles to maintain equilibrium. The initial diagnosis is based tentatively on the therapist's intense responses to the patient. Common feelings are of being "thrown," of walking on eggs, of being seduced and manipulated, but also of feeling like the best and most prized therapist in the world. The range and power of these responses helps therapists empathize with the disorganized and shifting attachment patterns of the BPD patient.

The immediate goal of the first few meetings is to keep the patient returning through development of the alliance. The therapist attempts to strike a middle ground of involvement so as to minimize the opportunity for extremes of idealization and devaluation and disorganization. The therapist must remember that the patient does not have a template for a cooperative reciprocal relationship and is expecting harm while hoping for unconditional love. Similarly, the patient has not developed the pragmatics of interpersonal language and cannot articulate her or his desires and hopes for the therapy. The patient enacts what she or he needs, wants, and fears. The therapist must translate the behaviors and respond to the underlying message.

Of central concern during the beginning stages of treatment is the reliability and availability of the therapist. The patient needs to experience the sturdy, safe, and reliable presence of the therapist, which involves establishing a structure and routine and offering consistent, kind responsiveness. An important aspect of this phase is educating the patient about the borderline disorder. This must be done in the terms and to the extent the patient can hear and understand. Psychoeducation about the disorder and how treatment works can provide needed structure and support. Also, during this phase it is important to attempt to engage family members who are still actively involved with the patient to provide education and determine whether family therapy is indicated.

During the initial sessions, the therapist is establishing the outline of a reciprocal relationship based on mutual respect and consideration. Also, the therapist is creating a structure within which inevitable disruptions and disappointments in the relationship can be discussed. This is a new experience for the patient, and it will take time for her or him to learn how to take advantage of this opportunity. The therapist discusses regular meeting times, crisis availability, referrals to a psychiatrist, and use of other resources. Negotiating with the patient is important, as the patient expects the therapist to exercise arbitrary authority.

Early on, the therapist will usually be pulled by the patient's neediness to set parameters that are either too rigid or too loose and erratic. When rigid limitations are set (e.g., no telephone calls between sessions, no assistance in obtaining additional resources), the patient will experience the therapist as unavailable and depriving despite her or his best efforts to comply. Not knowing how to ask for a different kind of help, the BPD patient may enact what she or he needs with provocative and self-destructive behaviors.

Although the patient may initially bond with the therapist who appears always to be available, the patient will not be able to evaluate when she or he is asking for too much and wearing down the therapist's goodwill. The therapist eventually becomes overburdened and is prone to either withdraw from the patient in subtle ways or suddenly set strict guidelines that threaten abandonment and prompt behavioral disorganization. This, in turn, reinforces the early experience of maltreatment and maintains maladaptive patterns.

In addition to negotiating the therapeutic framework, the therapist is determining how much and what kind of asylum and village the patient needs. The therapist organizes the treatment team and degree of structure needed in collaboration with the patient.

The recurrent issues and themes throughout treatment will be addressed in the next chapter. We now discuss general issues in termination and finish with a discussion of the therapeutic issues involved in psychopharmacological treatment.

TERMINATION OF TREATMENT

Children never outgrow their need for parents, although the nature and extent of the need and dependence shift throughout the life cycle. With this relational model in mind, the therapist considers with the patient what is needed to sustain optimal functioning given the patient's level of integration and environmental resources. The village that helped raise the child is still needed to sustain the adult.

As we have emphasized throughout this book, BPD patients require the opportunity for a dependent attachment over time to improve their functioning. Patients who have mild forms of the disorder may benefit from a 2- to 5-year course of psychotherapy, a more traditional termination process with the psychotherapist, and continued medication maintenance as needed. However, they too may return for treatment during life crises and to further rework developmental issues, as do many patients. Those with moderate forms of the disorder may benefit from "intermittent continuous" therapy over the life cycle, which is based on the medical model of a chronic disease with acute exacerbations (McGlashan 1993). Patients who have severe forms of the disorder will require a combination of ongoing case management, supportive psychotherapy, and medication maintenance, although with much less frequency and intensity. However, as Sylvia and Wendy have taught us (see Chapters 5 and 6, respectively), the need for a prosthetic form of treatment that wraps services around the patient so that they are in a continuous form of "life support" is ongoing.

As a general guideline, as the patient improves, the treatment team must be careful to maintain continued availability, within clear guidelines, as a sine qua non of the treatment. The more secure the patient feels that a safety net is available, the less need she or he will have for it. Although some clinicians may fear that this promotes a destructive dependency, the model proposed here and the case histories that illustrate it strongly support the importance of maintaining a solid and secure attachment base. Growth is sustained through maintenance of secure attachments. As patient and treatment team recognize the patient's increased stabilization and maturity, a weaning process of gradually reduced visits, treatment breaks, referral to therapy groups, and/or self-help groups in the community can be introduced. It is made clear that during times of crisis, a higher level of care is possible.

As challenging as work with BPD patients can be, it can also be among the most rewarding. Rarely in our work do we experience such dramatic improvement that is so closely related to the quality of our relationship with the patient. This work reaffirms our professional commitment to the psychotherapeutic process.

THERAPEUTIC ISSUES IN PHARMACOTHERAPY

Our focus in this section is with the psychotherapeutic issues that bear on pharmacotherapy for the BPD patient, not on the pharmacotherapy itself. For a review of medication strategies for treating BPD patients and a compendium of practical recommendations, the reader is referred to works by Stein (1992), Soloff (1993, 1994), and Gunderson (2001) and the American Psychiatric Association's (2001) *Practice Guideline for the Treatment of Patients With Borderline Personality Disorder.*

Although the primary treatment for patients with BPD is psychotherapy combined with a range of other mental health services, pharmacotherapy is a core component for the treatment of comorbid major depression, bipolar disorders, anxiety disorders, and paranoia and other transient psychotic states. It is also used to modulate affective lability even when the patient does not meet criteria for an Axis I disorder. However, as with all aspects of treatment, enlisting the patient's cooperation in pursuing the most appropriate course of medications is fraught with crisis and chaos. The challenge of pharmacotherapy is to enlist the patient's cooperation to take medications as prescribed and to provide accurate feedback regarding compliance and therapeutic side effects. If the therapist is also a psychiatrist, he or she may supply both medication and psychotherapy. More often, the therapist is a mental health professional who refers the patient to a physician experienced with psychopharmacological treatment.

Compliance with drug therapy is difficult for many but poses special problems for BPD patients. Although BPD patients readily self-medicate with alcohol and other illegal substances, they become the Ralph Nader of the U.S. Food and Drug Administration when advised to take prescription medicine. Worried about poisoning their body and being controlled by foreign substances, BPD patients may school themselves in the *Physicians' Desk Reference* and argue the risks rather than the benefits of the medication. BPD patients are often hypersensitive to medication effects despite their inordinately high pain tolerance to self-mutilation and overwork. Their concern is an extension of the hypervigilance about potential mistreatment by those in authority, especially caregivers, characteristic of BPD. They approach the relationship with the physician as they do all relationships, desperately wanting to trust and rely but fearing maltreatment. Because BPD patients lack a model of a cooperative relationship within which they can negotiate their needs and concerns, they feel at the mercy of the physician's perceived arbitrary power. Thus, the physician must focus as much attention on the alliance as on the best medication regimen.

When the therapist refers a BPD patient for medications, he or she often sparks fears of abandonment. The patient may also feel her or his problems are being minimized by a referral for a "pill" or worry that the therapist is incompetent and unable to provide care. These concerns need to be addressed and discussed openly when apparent. It is helpful to provide ongoing education about BPD and to point out that the disorder requires many different approaches simultaneously. Once the therapist determines that medications are indicated, the best approach to take with the BPD patient is a direct discussion of possible benefits of medication balanced by potential risks. The patient will need reassurance that the therapist is not abandoning her or him but plans continued involvement and that psychotherapy remains a core element.

A good professional marriage between physician and therapist is imperative for an effective team approach. Both partners need to respect and be supportive of each other and have open communication. Roles and responsibilities must be outlined for the patient, with the therapist maintaining the central relationship and the physician functioning as a collaborator and adjunctive figure. It is helpful to share similar views on the nature of the borderline disorder or at least on how to approach treatment. When differences or disagreements are too great, the patient may react through disruptive and dangerous behaviors, especially during times of crisis.

Under conditions of high stress and emotional arousal, and especially during disruptions in the alliance with either therapist or physician, patients will often turn to the therapist or physician to complain about the other. They will enlist support in getting their needs met from the disappointing other. When the therapist receives such a complaint about the physician, he or she must assist the patient in articulating what has transpired and coach the patient on how to discuss her concerns with the physician. Once the psychiatrist hears the patient's concerns, he or she must discuss them in as much detail as possible to assure the patient that he or she understands the patient's experience. The restoration of the therapeutic alliance through discussion and dialogue is a powerful learning experience for the patient in how to be direct and assertive about her or his needs. This facilitates the development of the use of pragmatic language.

Both therapist and physician can find themselves overselling the usefulness of medications to the recalcitrant patient and engaging in a struggle for control. Underneath the struggles often lies a fierce and naive wish that medications will magically cure the disorder. This wish is shared by both therapist and patient.

BPD patients often have very low tolerance for the physical discomfort of side effects because the discomfort increases their general level of dysphoria and they have not yet developed adequate distress tolerance skills. This can be puzzling to the therapist, as it stands in marked contrast to their high tolerance for self-induced pain. The latter usually occurs in a dissociative state that masks or dulls the acute sensation of pain. The empathic concern of the psychiatrist and therapist can help the patient tolerate the discomfort of side effects.

Comorbid Medical Conditions

Another complicating factor in both psychiatric and psychotherapeutic treatment is the presence of comorbid physical health problems. BPD patients often have pushed themselves too hard and have not attended to warning signs of physical strain and exhaustion. They also are susceptible to chronic pain syndromes, fibromyalgia, and chronic fatigue syndrome. Further, their overuse of drugs, alcohol, cigarettes, and food results in a range of health problems. Too often they do not comply with medical regimens for treatment of heart disease, diabetes, and other medical conditions, and their behaviors exacerbate these conditions. BPD patients often relate in a disorganized and unstable manner with all caregivers regardless of discipline. Their relational problems interfere with the establishment of a consistent working alliance with all health care professionals and impede proper diagnosis and treatment. Thus, the treating psychiatrist must work closely with other medical specialists to advocate for good medical care.

BPD patients may appear to exaggerate and amplify physical symptoms. This is related to their impaired ability to identify and label discrete emotional states. They lack an emotional vocabulary and may substitute the language of physical pain to describe both their physical and emotional suffering. It is also more acceptable to receive care for physical suffering. However, here too they have difficulty describing where they hurt in discrete terms, making it is hard to determine how medical and psychiatric conditions interact. However, with a persistent attitude of supportive inquiry, the patient can eventually improve her or his self-report of symptoms and side effects.

Alternative Forms of Healing

BPD patients are likely to seek out alternative forms of healing such as acupuncture, massage, chiropractic services, astrological forecasts, consultations with psychics, and herbal medicine. This stems from their general distrust of traditional authority figures and from their tendency to rely on alternative belief systems to understand the interpersonal world. Physician and therapist are most effective when encouraging all attempts at constructive self-care. These alternative methods, some of which are proving to be effective, are an additional means to modulate and regulate emotions and receive needed comfort and care. The patient, trusting that she or he is supported and respected in her or his efforts, will be more willing to experiment with medications.

Compliance

Once the patient agrees to try medications, the physician and therapist must work collaboratively to track efficacy and side effects. BPD patients rarely do what they are told. They will drink alcohol and take medications. They will experiment with increasing or decreasing the dosage, take medications intermittently, or discontinue them suddenly. Their compliance problems stem from poor self-monitoring capacity, low frustration tolerance, and a general mistrust of those in authority. They become easily discouraged and hopeless. Periodically, BPD patients will stop medications to make themselves worse and push themselves to the edge of misery—a strategy, like cutting, that is aimed toward relief. Noncompliance can be used as a form of protest and communication when life crises occur or the therapeutic relationship falters. The psychiatrist above all else needs to maintain the alliance with the patient and view these behaviors as part of the disorder and as forms of communication. Active collaboration with treatment team members can provide needed support and sustenance.

Substance Abuse

Another challenge facing the psychiatrist is how to manage co-occurring substance abuse disorders. There is a growing body of research on treatment of dual disorders that supports an integrated approach that combines psychiatric interventions with drug treatment and relapse and recovery strategies (Drake et al. 1998; Judd et al. 2002; Minkoff, 2001a, 2001b). Guidelines are also being established for pharmacotherapy with dually diagnosed patients (Albanese 2001). In general, it appears that it may be more effective to treat psychiatric conditions with medications even while the patient continues to abuse drugs and alcohol. Although this may pose ethical concerns for the psychiatrist, there is a growing body of evidence to suggest that it is a calculated risk worth taking.

REFERENCES

Albanese MJ: Assessing and treating comorbid mood and substance use disorders. Psychiatric Times 18(4):55–57, 2001

Allness DJ, Knoedler WH: The PACT Model of Community-Based Treatment for Persons With Severe and Persistent Mental Illnesses: A Manual for PACT Start-Up. Arlington, VA, NAMI Anti-Stigma Foundation, 1998

American Psychiatric Association: Practice guideline for the treatment of patients with borderline personality disorder. Am J Psychiatry 158 (10, suppl):1–52, 2001

Berkowitz CB, Gunderson JG: Multifamily psychoeducational treatment of borderline personality disorder, in Multifamily Groups in the Treatment of Severe Psychiatric Disorders. Edited by McFarlane WR, Lefley HP. New York, Guilford, 2002, pp 268–290

Bernstein E, Putnam F: Development, reliability, and validity of a dissociation scale. J Nerv Ment Dis 174:727–735, 1986

Bernstein DP, Fink L, Handelsman L, et al: Initial reliability and validity of a new retrospective measure of child abuse and neglect. Am J Psychiatry 151: 1132–1136, 1994

Bowlby J: Attachment and Loss, Vol 1: Attachment (1969). New York, Basic Books, 1982

Bowlby J: A Secure Base: Parent-Child Attachment and Healthy Human Development. New York, Basic Books, 1988

Brooner RK, Herbst JH, Schmidt CW: Antisocial personality disorder among drug abusers: relations to other personality diagnoses and the five-factor model of personality. J Nerv Ment Dis 181:313–319, 1993

Clarkin JF, Kernberg OF, Yeomans F: Psychotherapy for Borderline Personality. New York, Wiley, 1999

Clarkin JF, Foelsch PA, Levy KN, et al: The development of a psychodynamic treatment for patients with borderline personality disorder: a preliminary study of behavioral change. Journal of Personality Disorders 15:487–495, 2001

Drake E, Merer-McFadden C, Mueser K, et al: Review of integrated mental health and substance abuse treatment for patients with dual disorders. Schizophr Bull 24:589–603, 1998

Fyer MR, Frances AJ, Sullivan T, et al: Comorbidity of borderline personality disorder. Arch Gen Psychiatry 45:348–352, 1988

Gunderson JG: Borderline Personality Disorder: A Clinical Guide. Washington, DC, American Psychiatric Publishing, 2001

Helzer JE, Pryzbeck TR: The co-occurrence of alcoholism with other psychiatric disorders in the general population and its impact on treatment. J Stud Alcohol 49:219–224, 1988

Hoffman P: Family intervention: DBT family skills training. Presentation at the Sixth International Congress on Disorders of Personality, Geneva, Switzerland, September 1999

Hoffman PD, Hooley JM: Expressed emotion and the treatment of borderline personality disorder. In Session 4(3):39–54, 1998

Judd P, Thomas N, Hough RL: UCSD/San Diego County Dual Diagnosis Demonstration Project: a prospective study of long-term outcomes and cost-benefits. Poster presentation at the Academy of Health Services Research and Health Policy Annual Research Meeting, Washington, DC, June 25, 2002

Keller H: The Story of My Life. New York, Doubleday, Page, 1903

Lezak MD: Neuropsychological Assessment, 2nd Edition. New York, Oxford University Press, 1983

Linehan MM: Cognitive-Behavioral Treatment of Borderline Personality Disorder. New York, Guilford, 1993a

Linehan MM: Skills Training Manual for Treating Borderline Personality Disorder. New York, Guilford, 1993b

Linehan MM: Understanding Borderline Personality Disorder. New York, Guilford, 1995

Linehan MM, Heard HL, Armstrong HE: Naturalistic follow-up of a behavioral treatment for chronically parasuicidal borderline patients. Arch Gen Psychiatry 50:971–974, 1993

Linehan MM, Tutek DA, Heard HL, et al: Interpersonal outcome of cognitive behavioral treatment for chronically suicidal borderline patients. Am J Psychiatry 151:1771–1776, 1994

Links PS, Heslegrave RJ, Mitton JE, et al: Borderline personality disorder and substance abuse: consequences of co-morbidity. Can J Psychiatry 40:9–14, 1995

McGlashan T: The Chestnut Lodge Follow-Up Study, Part III: long-term outcome of borderline personalities. Arch Gen Psychiatry 42:20–30, 1986

McGlashan TH: Implications of outcome research for the treatment of borderline personality disorder, in Borderline Personality Disorder: Etiology and Treatment. Edited by Paris J. Washington, DC, American Psychiatric Press, 1993, pp 235–260

Meloy JR: Prediction of violence in outpatient psychotherapy. Am J Psychother 41:38–45, 1987

Milner B: Inter-hemispheric differences in the localization of psychological processes in man. Br Med Bull 27:272–277, 1971

Minkoff K: Developing standards of care for individuals with co-occurring psychiatric and substance use disorders. Psychiatr Serv 52:597–599, 2001a

Minkoff K: Program components of a comprehensive integrated care system for seriously mentally ill patients with substance disorders. New Dir Ment Health Serv 91:17–30, 2001b

Money J: The Standardized Road-Map Test of Direction Sense. San Rafael, CA, Academic Therapy Publications, 1976

Osterreith PA: Le test de cople d'une figure complexe. Archive de Psychologie 30:206–356, 1944

Poling J, Rounsaville BJ, Ball S, et al: Rates of personality disorders in substance abusers. Journal of Personality Disorders 13:375–384, 1999

Ruff R, Light RH, Evans R: The Ruff Figural Fluency Test: a normative study with adults. Developmental Neuropsychology 3:37–51, 1987

Soloff PH: Pharmacological therapies in borderline personality disorder, in Borderline Personality Disorder: Etiology and Treatment. Edited by Paris J. Washington, DC, American Psychiatric Press, 1993, pp 319–348

Soloff PH: Is there any drug treatment of choice for the borderline patient? Acta Psychiatr Scand 89:50–55, 1994

Stein G: Drug treatment of the personality disorders. Br J Psychiatry 161:167–184, 1992

Stone MH, Hurt SW, Stone DK: The P.I.-500: long-term follow-up of borderline in-patients meeting DSM-III criteria, I: global outcome. Journal of Personality Disorders 1:291–298, 1987

Tyrer P, Gunderson J, Lyons M, et al: Extent of comorbidity between mental state and personality disorders (special feature). Journal of Personality Disorders 11:242–259, 1997

Wechsler DA: A standardized memory scale for clinical use. J Psychol 19:87–95, 1945

Wechsler DA: The Measurement and Appraisal of Adult Intelligence, 4th Edition. Baltimore, MD, Williams & Wilkins, 1958

Weschler D: Wechsler Adult Intelligence Scale—Revised Manual. New York, Psychological Corporation/Harcourt, Brace, Jovanovich, 1981

Winnicott DW: The Maturational Process and the Facilitating Environment. London, Hogarth Press, 1965

Witkin HA, Oltman PK, Raskin E, et al: A Manual of the Embedded Figures Tests. Palo Alto, CA, Consulting Psychology Press, 1971

Recurrent Themes and Issues

Do unto others as you would have them do unto you.

The Golden Rule

From home a banished city…
…the presence of that absence is everywhere

Edna St. Vincent Millay

The limits of my language are the limits of my world.

Ludwig Wittgenstein

In the last chapter, we discussed the universal elements of treatment. In this final chapter, we elaborate on the phenomenology of the disorder from the perspective of the developmental model as a means to inform treatment. We review the recurrent themes and issues that challenge therapists in their work with BPD patients, with an emphasis on deepening our understanding of the patient's experience. The sections are organized roughly according to the major domains of clinical phenomenology—intense unstable relationships, cognitive dysfunction, emotional and behavioral dysregulation—even though they are like woof and warp and deeply embedded with one another.

The multiple states of mind regarding attachment that characterize BPD are enacted with the therapist and treatment team. As such, BPD patients provide a striking example of how, in daily life, humans generally do unto others as they have been done to. A major goal of treatment is to restore the Golden Rule to the course of their human relationships

through stabilizing and integrating these states of mind and, in so doing, bringing greater stability to their identity and relationships. In this
chapter, we highlight the multiple models or states of mind regarding
attachment that BPD patients exhibit, the challenges each presents for
the treatment team, and general treatment strategies. We also address common issues within the therapeutic relationship. We begin with a brief
discussion of empathy, as it is so central to the therapeutic work.

EMPATHY

BPD patients' empathic capacity varies considerably depending on the
severity of the disorder. Among different states of mind, their empathic
ability fluctuates according to their state of mind. When not emotionally involved in a situation, most BPD patients can employ empathy—
some to a high degree. Once they are threatened or in an intense state
of need, however, their analytic abilities disappear and they become
highly self-centered, concrete, and context bound. These fluctuations
throw the therapist off and interfere with his or her empathic capacity
toward the patient. It is a challenge to maintain empathy toward a person who is not empathic with others, especially when that person mis-
understands, devalues, and attacks.

As discussed in Chapter 1 (see "Metacognitive Monitoring"), empathy is a highly developed mental capacity and an endpoint of interpersonal cognitive development. It represents the capacity to "put one's
self in another person's shoes" and arrive at an understanding of his
or her experience. This highly abstract yet unconscious process requires
sophisticated analytic and synthetic abilities. It requires the self to take
into account the situation-specific features of the present context with a
historic knowledge of the other's unique properties (e.g., temperament,
intelligence, gender, religious background) and to compare and contrast
these against one's own history and experience. It requires a decentered
analysis. Empathic capacity may be part of our genetic heritage as an
important means of survival. For full development, it appears to require the experience of our intentions being understood and responded
to by significant others in a consistent manner.

Work with BPD patients requires a better than average ability to maintain consistent empathy, since the patient fails in this endeavor toward
herself or himself, the therapist, and important others. The solo thera-
pist/psychiatrist and treatment team will require continuous opportunities to discuss and review their work so as to maintain an empathic
stance. Before clinicians can help BPD patients develop more consistent

empathy, they themselves must have an environment within which to obtain needed support and understanding for the challenges of working with BPD patients. This can be accomplished by regular clinical supervision and consultation on an individual or group basis as well as continuing education programs. We believe it is potentially dangerous and certainly anxiety-provoking to work with BPD patients without strong collegial support and consultation.

INTENSE UNSTABLE RELATIONSHIPS

Idealization and Falling in Love With the Therapist

BPD patients learned that tending to parents' needs provided them with an island of safety and attention, a quasi-secure attachment, in an otherwise unpredictable, depriving, or harsh environment. Caretaking may have taken the form of emotional tending, cooking, homemaking, nursing, sexualized physical contact, or actual sexual involvement. Although this precocious caretaking extracted a high price, it also helped the BPD patient develop capacities and skills. Among these are loyalty, discipline, and responsibility. This caretaking relationship with the parent(s) formed the basis for the preoccupied attachment model that we speculate serves as the template for the establishment of the therapeutic relationship and enables the BPD patient to engage in therapy. As the patient enters treatment, she brings with her a readiness to attach in a devoted and compliant manner. She longs to admire and love the therapist and feel the same in return. The therapist must be willing and able to tolerate this initial devotion and idealization, because it enables the patient to form an alliance. However, numerous pitfalls and ethical dilemmas accompany this process.

One of the many aspects missing from the BPD patient's early relationships is the experience of loving the parent freely in the purely innocent form that children display. There is usually a coercive aspect to the relationship, and the patient must conform to parental needs. When a 3-year-old picks a flower for his mother with great pleasure and pride and she responds with pleasure and delight, the child learns how to love and give. When the parent commands the child to pick the flower or repeatedly ignores or criticizes the gift, he feels deflated and shamed, inadequate, and unlovable.

The therapeutic relationship offers the opportunity to learn how to relate in a noncoercive way. The patient may bring in gifts such as writings, artwork, articles, or small presents. The therapist must keep in mind that the BPD patient was probably unable to give and express love to parents in a spontaneous fashion and have her or his love appreciated and valued. Rather than interpret these behaviors, the therapist is wise to accept them graciously and with appreciation. Should the patient overdo these behaviors, as she or he overdoes many others, and offer something too expensive or personal, the therapist can discuss the multiple meanings of the gift. It is at this point that a discussion of professional ethics can take place. More valuable, however, may be a discussion of how it feels to be given something that is too much or too personal a gift. The patient learns more by direct discussion of these issues than by falling back on a rigid reading of the ethics code.

Many BPD patients develop a crush or fall in love with their therapist or a member of the treatment team. These feelings can become sexualized. In most forms of psychotherapy, the standard approach is to explore these feelings. With the BPD patient, this must be approached carefully depending on the severity of the disorder and the patient's history of sexual abuse. An assessment must be made as to the developmental level it represents. Some patients describe an adolescent crush, whereas others describe a fantasy of a sexual relationship and marriage. Still others can only become involved in a relationship by sexualizing it. Some patients, for example, demand a sexual relationship as the only way the therapist can prove his or her interest.

In general, it is most helpful for the therapist to accept the patient's expressions of being "in love" as real and understandable given the uniqueness of the therapeutic relationship and the absence of unconditional and respectful love in the patient's childhood. The opportunity to have these feelings acknowledged without rejection or punishment is a new experience for the patient. Interpretation of the behavior in a manner that makes the patient feel wrong for having the feelings will be experienced as a rejection and blaming. At the same time, the therapist must reinforce the professional and safe aspects of the relationship. The challenge for the therapist is to tolerate the intensity of the patient's emotion without pushing her away or pulling her too close. Consultation and collegial support are essential during these times. The therapist must first find his or her own balance and then work to understand the patient's behavior and how best to respond so both therapist and patient are protected and can continue the therapeutic work.

Of special concern is a sexual or other exploitative relationship between therapist and patient. Because BPD patients are so hungry to attach to strong caregiving figures and have poorly developed personal limits, they are at great risk for exploitation by therapists, ministers, physicians, and employers who are needy and disturbed. As adults, BPD patients may tolerate considerable misuse by others to whom they feel devoted. BPD patients who were sexually abused as children are especially at risk for sexual involvement with the therapist or others in positions of trust. Similarly, BPD patients can be exploited in work and volunteer positions, as they will overwork. They can be blind-sighted by their great neediness and desire to be special into believing that the person in authority has their best interests at heart. Conversely, if these patients feel betrayed, they can falsely accuse the therapist or team member of sexual involvement as a means to avenge themselves and fight back. BPD patients can shift quickly from victim to victimizer.

Devaluation, Splitting, and Manipulation

When BPD patients feel deprived, betrayed, or victimized, they experience anger and anxiety that activates coercive and controlling attachment behaviors. The significant other who is apparently triggering this state is viewed, at worst, as an enemy and, at best, as withholding. During these states, the patient employs "splitting," which is a manifestation of preoperational thinking. It reflects an inability to think dichotomously—that is, to entertain opposing feelings and thoughts about a person and understand that he or she has complex motivations. At this preoperational level of cognitive and emotional development, the patient uses attributes of the other idiosyncratically to represent the whole person and reacts to these with one-dimensional and pervasive emotions that have an either-or quality (Lane and Schwartz 1987). The patient interprets the surface responses and characteristics of the team member as depriving, mean, and withholding.

BPD patients can be expert at manipulation, intimidation, and bullying. Even though these behaviors appear to push the treatment team away, they are designed to pull the team close so that the patient can get his or her needs met, reduce anxiety, and restore equilibrium. These behaviors are the ones that animals in the wild employ to survive; they are required to stave off attackers, find food, and preserve habitat. Normally developing toddlers use these strategies until they learn that other means are more socially effective. BPD patients were often coerced as children and learned to do this to others.

When the patient has a treatment team—that is, more than one clinician—the patient will complain to one team member about how badly she or he is being treated by another team member. This can instigate conflict between or among team members over how best to care for the patient. The conflict usually divides the treatment team into the "tough love" and "mother love" camps. The tough love group feels that the patient needs greater limit setting, whereas the mother love group believes that the patient needs greater understanding and support. The tough love group feels the mother love group is reinforcing the manipulative behavior of the patient, while the mother love group feels they are providing needed treatment.

The challenge for the team is to collaborate with the patient in understanding the behavior and determining her or his needs. The first step is to apply a developmental perspective. Children learn which parent is more likely to meet their immediate needs. They can resort to temper tantrums or disorganized behaviors when these needs are not met. Under conditions of deprivation and threat, BPD patients' tenuous trust and connection to the team member is broken; they are once again deprived toddlers fighting alone in desperation.

Such behavior usually reflects a perception of the situation that is partially accurate. It usually occurs when one team member is feeling anxious, helpless, and resentful and is pushed beyond his emotional resources and/or has countertransference responses such as feeling he is struggling with his own coercive parents. The result is a rigid and punitive response to the patient under the guise of limit setting to regain control and emotional equilibrium. Conversely, the team member who appears overly solicitous of the patient may be operating from the opposite countertransference position—for example, wishing she had received more parental understanding and support.

The patient in a bullying and coercive state of mind often surprises the therapist. It is difficult to extend understanding of the immaturity of the BPD patients when they appear otherwise of reasonable intelligence and competence. Their "good" functioning or "apparent competence" (Linehan 1993a, 1995) crumbles dramatically under interpersonal stress.

During such states, it is important for team members to discuss the patient's concerns and to hear the message behind the breast-beating, because this is the primary method for reducing anxiety. Also, the patient must believe that recourse is available when the relationship with any team member feels untenable. Most BPD patients had no one to turn to as a buffer or protector from maltreating parents. It is important that this lonely and desperate state not be re-created in the treatment setting. There must be hope for getting needs met.

Abandonment

The fear of abandonment is a central concern for BPD patients. Their inner state is that of the lone ravenous wolf. They often fight and avoid dependence on others, but once attached, they feel overwhelmingly dependent. These patients, when feeling abandoned, have the experience of being "thrown away" as though they were an infant left in the parking lot, discarded in the most careless and callous manner. There is no shelter in their world. It is this state of utter helplessness, adrift and alone, to which the therapist must attend. Wendy (see Chapter 6) captured this with heartrending clarity when she wrote in her letter to her therapist, "Everybody leaves me . . . as if I dropped from the skies . . . how much I have longed to have parents and a home . . . "

BPD patients' response to feelings of aloneness and abandonment are related to the absence of a secure attachment mode and of what has been termed "evocative memory" (Adler and Buie 1979). *Evocative memory* refers to the ability to remember the soothing and comforting features of a secure, loving relationship and to recall that help is available and reliable. As discussed by Gunderson (1996), without evocative memories of secure attachment, BPD patients are highly dependent on real care from others for reassurance of proximity and sense of safety. The retrieval of an attachment mode is context bound and requires certain affective states for activation. In a state of distress, whatever soothing and loving memories the BPD patient may have experienced cannot be retrieved because they are dissociated and stored in a separate memory system. Even more likely, they were never encoded or are too fragmented to retrieve. Instead, the patient experiences the presence of absence, a state devoid of human connection that induces anxiety and dysphoria.

We emphasize that the experience of abandonment can become a life-and-death matter. The patient feels she or he cannot survive without the relationship. Once the therapist and team realize this, appropriate team structures and routines are established to provide a constant experience of the reliable presence and availability. These include regular appointments, clear policies on crisis availability, coverage during vacation, and after-hours availability.

Anxiety Over Improvement

BPD patients do not often report progress, happy moments, or successes. The tenacity to report what is wrong with their life is frustrating and discouraging to the therapist. The patient appears to amplify every complaint, whether it is related to mood, physical pain, or a life event. Wanting to be helpful and to see progress, the therapist may point out successes that the patient has not yet experienced as such. Instead of feeling supported, she feels misunderstood and pushed away. She fears that the therapist is really saying, "You no longer need me." In response, the patient may complain louder or, worse, enact how badly she feels through self-destructive behavior in order to prove she still requires help.

We draw a parallel to the description in Chapter 1 ("An Integrated Developmental Model") of preoccupied attachment, in which the child cannot calm down or attend to play because he does not trust that the mother will return and care for him. Thus, he focuses on the mother by emitting signs of continuous distress. Until the patient develops a more stable attachment, he will require reminders that the team is available. The patient fears being cast adrift, a replication of his childhood experience.

The patient does need validation for accomplishments through encouragement, praise, and admiration from the therapist, but it must be related to current developmental accomplishments. The challenge for the therapist is to acknowledge maturation as it manifests itself while emphasizing that therapeutic support and work will continue as long as the patient needs it.

Secrecy

BPD patients report daily events and historical information in fragments and often withhold critical pieces of information. Early in treatment they are unable to elaborate about interpersonal events and can rarely give a detailed description of an encounter. It feels to the therapist as though they are keeping secrets or consciously withholding information. This secret information ranges from successes at work and school to substance abuse and sexual relationships. Sexual secrets are especially common among patients who have been involved in incestuous relationships or when sexual behavior was the focus of particular scorn and disapproval by the parents. Susan exemplifies the role of secrecy in BPD patients through her secret affair with a former Chestnut Lodge aide (see Chapter 4).

Secret promiscuous sexual activity, as illustrated in the cases of Lillian and Susan (see Chapters 3 and 4, respectively), forms part of a highly fragmented preverbal attachment schema. The patient may engage in sexual behaviors in a dissociated fashion as a means to restore feeling or, depending on the context, avoid and numb feelings. When the sexual activity serves its function of emotional regulation, the sexual partner may be demeaned or discarded as though the activity itself is disowned.

BPD patients fear that disclosure of secrets will spoil their pleasure. The manner in which their enjoyable activities and moments were ruined is often heartbreaking and instructive. Sharing information about the self places one at risk, and silence is a great protector. Their theory is that what others do not know can hurt neither them nor the other. Susan realized that informing staff of her involvement with the former Chestnut Lodge aide would result in an admonition to end the relationship.

Also, we suspect that BPD patients do not readily share accomplishments because they do not expect an admiring response. As an example, the persistence with which Susan's father labeled her as "dumb" must have undermined her academic efforts. Certainly, she would not have readily brought home even minor evidence of success fearing further ridicule. Also, in the black-and-white thinking characteristic of BPD patients, success and need for treatment cannot coexist. Continued availability of support is contingent on the continuous expression of distress.

Secrecy can also serve as an expression of maturation and developmental achievement. It is a part of normal development to keep some activities private and out of the purview of parents. We all must learn that honesty is not always the best policy and that too much information can cause unnecessary hurt. The ability to be discrete, keep information to ourselves, and protect our own and others' privacy implies a sense of a self who has a private life and can share or withhold information on the basis of its social impact and consequences.

Constructing an Autobiography

An important part of the therapeutic work is developing a life narrative, not as an end in itself, but as a means to elaborate and integrate multiple attachment models. Fragmentation and dissociation have prevented the construction of a coherent biography. When the patient is asked to provide a chronological history that integrates biographical facts with attendant emotions, confusion and chaos result. The therapist must help the patient generate explanations about her or his life, not through open inquiry as in free association but through a combination of education and highly structured reflection. There is great variability in the extent to which this can actually be accomplished, and it is based on the degree and magnitude of biological vulnerability and maltreatment. We first present what is possible for patients with mild to moderate forms of the disorder and then discuss how this approach can be modified for patients with serious impairment.

Psychoeducation is an important feature of treatment. First, all patients can be educated to varying degrees of sophistication about how their particular temperament, trait, and cognitive vulnerabilities contributed to the disorder. Similarly, they can be taught how their vulnerabilities may have interacted with the personality and temperament of family members and adverse life events to create their unique strengths and problems. This entails helping patients understand how these multiple interactions fostered and hindered their development in relationships, emotional and behavioral regulation, and self-esteem. Patients who have mild to moderate impairment can be helped to understand how they generate interactions with others on the basis of early learning that repeats the experience of maltreatment and how they may now perpetuate unsatisfying outcomes.

This emotionally based educational process can take place through individual psychotherapy alone, psychosocial rehabilitative strategies, or a combination of psychotherapy and a structured group psychoeducational format as developed by Linehan (1993a, 1993b). This educational process is different from psychotherapy with healthier non-BPD patients who have a more well integrated attachment model and can gradually discover and uncover this information with less assistance from the therapist. BPD patients lack this organization and require a more active construction of their biography in the context of active treatment.

The treatment team must realize that the construction of a biography is both comforting and threatening to the patient. It allows her to make sense of her behavior and to understand why she has such enormous difficulty in relationships and tolerating emotions. It reduces her intense self-blame while strengthening her ability to accept responsibility for her actions. It also builds greater understanding of the behavior of family members. At the same time, the patient must face sad truths about her family and her self.

At the most extreme end of the maltreatment spectrum, the patient may realize that she was, perhaps, unloved and treated with complete disregard for her needs, such as in the case of Wendy (see Chapter 6). This feeling of being a "motherless child" carries a sense of overwhelming aloneness in the world, and nothing truly makes up for the early absences. It is devastating to learn that the people you depended on so desperately were inadequate to the task. It is also difficult to accept that you have perpetuated problems through misreading interpersonal situations in a manner too narrow and personalized or that you have may have hurt others and been abusive yourself.

However, the experience with the treatment team, when new, helps the patient construct an identity as a more worthwhile person, one who makes mistakes from which one can learn. As this understanding unfolds, the patient is able to process larger segments of biographical memory into a more integrated whole. The patient with more impairment will process and integrate this information to a far more limited degree, if at all, but will improve through the containment provided by the supportive treatment network.

COGNITIVE DYSFUNCTION

Dissociation

As elaborated earlier, pathological dissociation underlies the inadequate cognitive and emotional integration of biographical information. BPD patients live much of their waking life in a trancelike state of disconnection from their own emotions. Consciousness, or the "feeling of what happens" (Damasaio 1999), is absent in a dissociative state. The patient does not experience the emotions that generate links among interpersonal events and models of attachment. Patients will describe "going blank" or "being spacey" during or following a significant event or within the therapy. This constitutes the experience of depersonalization and derealization. Without attendant emotions, we do not feel real, nor do our experiences seem real. Similarly, emotions surprise the patient and trigger a shift in state of mind during the session. The interconnections between emotion and trigger are missing or not activated to create a rich, complex picture of an interpersonal encounter and to experience the self across situations. BPD patients cannot construct emotional causation and consequences.

As will be discussed in greater detail later in this section, dissociation disappears or diminishes as the patient learns to identify and discriminate among emotional states and link them to interpersonal triggers. As the patient develops a language about her or his emotional experiences and improves emotional coding and decoding, the patient's overall cognitive abilities can mature. Splitting, denial, and projection diminish or disappear and are replaced by more complex interpersonal analysis. The extent to which this is possible is determined by the severity of the cognitive processing problems and the severity of child maltreatment.

Use of Language

Another aspect of the BPD cognitive problem is poor development of pragmatic language, or the use of words and phrases that initiate and sustain a conversation so that a need-satisfying relationship can be formed. Also, BPD patients have a poorly developed emotional vocabulary to describe their internal state.

In treatment, this translates to a marked absence of "flow." It is difficult to settle into a predictable rhythm, as BPD patients lack a consistent modus operandi both within and between sessions. Silence is followed by disorganized and fragmented speech followed by telegraphic statements. This reflects poor language development and the underlying multiple state shifts and disorganized attachment schemas.

BPD patients are often blunt, sometimes crude, and opinionated and are known for calling "a spade, a spade." They lose social context and can be brutally honest about others' weaknesses and their own behaviors. Their honesty is frequently misinterpreted as mean spirited and devaluing or provocative and manipulative. However, these patients are calling it as they see it without full analysis of the interpersonal consequences. They lack social finesse and are concrete in their communications.

Alternately, when there is disruption in the therapeutic relationship or the session has triggered painful memories, BPD patients may become silent and the "speechless child" emerges. They appear disconnected or guarded and menacing, yet are also in a dissociated state and unable to voice what they appear to be feeling. During these moments, the therapist attempts to articulate what the patient might be experiencing. In this way, words bring meaning and organization to inchoate experience, and the patient begins to develop her or his own vocabulary.

A frequent presentation of language is that of a disorganized waterfall of words that do not cohere. Sentence and paragraph structure are awry. This usually occurs when the patient is attempting to explain emotionally arousing interpersonal events. The therapist strains to understand the patient's syntax and interpersonal logic. Many BPD patients also use words imprecisely and become confused by metaphors and sayings. They are unsure of the meanings of words or experience words as powerless to impact others. These difficulties partially arise from the absence of dialogue about thoughts and feelings and the contradictory manner in which words were used in their families; affect was incongruent with message.

For BPD patients with diagnosed learning disabilities, language impairment may be even greater and related to poor auditory processing of words and limited verbal fluency. These patients have difficulty translating what has been said and formulating a response. This problem with "thinking on their feet" is amplified under conditions of high stress as emotion further disorganizes already faulty processing abilities.

Cognitive Distortions

One of the most common and debilitating features of the borderline disorder is distorted interpretation of interpersonal situations. Although BPD patients hear what others say, their emotional experience of the message short-circuits their ability to process the whole message in its social context. Thinking is hijacked by emotion. This creates frequent disruptions in treatment and social situations.

These distortions are related to the cognitive operations of denial and splitting described earlier and results in the black-and-white, good-or-bad, all-or-nothing thinking style so characteristic of BPD patients. Because BPD patients are unable to apply metacognitive monitoring and knowledge, they make frequent errors in interpreting interpersonal behavior. They apply a narrow paranoid lens or accept surface attributes with passive naiveté. Wendy provides numerous extreme examples of this problem as she attacked her therapists verbally and physically misinterpreted their intentions (see Chapter 6). Another example is of a patient recently hospitalized for burning herself. Frightened and mistrustful of staff and patients on the ward, she struck up a quick friendship with a severely antisocial patient, believing his superficial glibness was genuine caring. She soon began talking about marrying him as a means of solving multiple problems postdischarge.

Hypervigilance, Odd Thinking, and Overvalued Ideas

BPD patients swing from a state of naive trust to bewilderment and confusion to paranoia about human motivations and behaviors. A general suspiciousness about the actions and motives of others colors their interpersonal world. The BPD patient has learned to be hypervigilant to interpersonal cues to manage anxiety and guard against potential harm. Maltreated children learn to watch for signs that they might be hurt. Maltreated children with cognitive and emotional deficits must develop even greater alertness. Parents were often so unpredictable and the child so unable to discriminate among their behaviors that only continuous attention afforded a modicum of protection.

Hypervigilance is apparent in the therapeutic relationship as BPD patients scan the therapist's face and note any physical changes in the room to determine how safe the session will be. They have exquisite sensitivity to any change; it signals potential threat and fear. Hypervigilance also underlies the belief in a sixth sense or telepathic ability in which some BPD patients believe. Because they cannot rely on a psychological understanding of human behavior, they turn to parapsychological theories such as astrology and tarot. Lillian took up astrology during the follow-up period, indicating continued mystification by the interpersonal world (see Chapter 3).

BPD patients frequently misinterpret others' behaviors as signs and portents of harm and abuse. Sylvia and Wendy repeatedly misinterpreted their therapists' interpretations and behaviors in this manner. One patient, Ann, while hospitalized for medical problems (an especially difficult experience for BPD patients), was convinced that the nurses and doctors were conspiring to give her poor care. In reality, she had been diagnosed with cancer and they were attempting to protect her from the emotional impact of the diagnosis. She identified correctly that something was amiss but arrived at the wrong conclusion. Her misinterpretation caused her to behave badly toward the staff and eventually receive the bad care she feared.

The reverse of mistrust is a naive and idealistic belief in the integrity of others. BPD patients have overvalued ideas about justice, honor, and duty in tandem with their distrust. They lack an appreciation for the complex gradations in motive and meaning of human behavior. This springs from their immature moral developmental and their enormous wish for a safe dependence on others. These beliefs offer hope in an otherwise threatening world. Concepts of competition, envy, and jealousy are poorly developed. Consequently, BPD patients are often bitterly disappointed when they encounter these "baser" motivations in others. Instead of seeing them as merely human, the patient attributes far more malevolence, typically meanness and exploitation. Therapeutic work focuses repeatedly on seeing the "gray" areas in self and others so that the patient can understand and accept the full range of human feelings and motivations.

Transient Paranoid States

The underlying cognitive vulnerabilities of BPD are most pronounced under conditions that combine extreme threat, high anxiety, loss or abandonment, and depression. These emotional states interfere with fluid and flexible processing of interpersonal information for everyone. However, for BPD patients, these conditions pose a critical danger, and their response is often rigidly paranoid. Their paranoia can assume delusional proportions for brief periods of time. No one in the patient's life is immune to becoming the paranoid object under these conditions. In this state, the patient can be dangerous and potentially homicidal, suicidal, or both. On a lesser scale, lawsuits and malpractice claims are filed during these periods.

The paranoid view enables one, in the short term, to mobilize resources for survival. Thus, it is fruitless to challenge these beliefs when the patient is acutely paranoid. Rather, the goal is to decrease emotional arousal by empathizing with the patient's feeling of threat and alarm and helping her or him take prosocial action to protect the self. This does not mean that the therapist validates the reality of the fear but that the therapist conveys understanding as to why the patient feels as she or he does given her or his construction of the situation.

Environmental interventions are usually essential. For example, when the paranoid object is a co-worker, a letter indicating the need for time off from work can provide the patient with distance and a cooling-off period. Medications to treat anxiety and paranoid thinking are indicated. When homicidal plans are mobilized, it may be necessary to hospitalize the patient, notify legal authorities, and warn intended victims.

Other Transient Psychotic States

During major depressive episodes exacerbated by loss or abandonment, or during periods of high stress, the cognitive functioning of BPD patients may further collapse. BPD patients are vulnerable to depression with psychotic features. These psychotic states usually take the form of hearing voices of significant others telling them they are no good and should die. They may also hear voices of parents or significant others that are critical or demeaning or occasionally comforting. Wendy persistently heard voices of three people admonishing or advising her.

Patients also report psychotic-like experiences that mirror maltreatment by parents, such as being hit, yelled at, or touched sexually. Sylvia was haunted by illusions of her dead mother sitting in her rocking chair and smells of her perfume. Other psychotic or altered states can occur when memories of particularly traumatic events are recalled. Sylvia developed paralysis of her legs when discussing her father's confession of sexual misdeeds. Wendy attacked her therapist violently when reminded of her drunken father falling on her in bed.

EMOTIONAL DYSREGULATION

A major challenge in working with BPD patients concerns their affective instability. Their emotional responses, on the surface, seem out of all proportion. They alternate between hypersensitivity and insensitivity to others. They have an exaggerated response to life's miseries and a dulled response to life's pleasures or an apparent absence of emotional response when one is most expected. It is difficult to read accurately their emotional expressions and determine what they need. They beat their chest when they want love and cut themselves when hurt and angry.

The therapeutic situation seeks to modify this developmental problem. The therapist helps the patient to decode emotions and learn emotional causation through the development of a shared meaning for language. Language accrues meaning as the patient experiences the congruence of the therapist's emotions, behaviors, and words with her or his own. Music, rhythm, and step must match for a fluid dance.

Just as each parent-child dyad develops their own pattern of relating that contains both universal and idiosyncratic elements, so must therapist and patient. The therapeutic task is to help the patient learn how to identify emotions and treat them as information and signals for adaptive behavior. The therapist learns to interpret the patient's behaviors as signs of discomfort, fear, pain, or pleasure and to respond through action and tone of voice in a manner that amplifies or modifies the patient's response. As the therapist accurately reads and mirrors the patient's signals, the feeling is modulated.

For example, during critical periods in the toddler stage, children become upset when mother leaves the room. Mother acknowledges this emotion and assists the child in tolerating it by stating in a reassuring tone of voice as she leaves the room, "I'll be back soon," while physically comforting the child. When she returns and says, "I'm back," with a hug, the child is reassured of mother's reliability. The voicing of the word "soon" gradually assumes symbolic meaning for the child so that he or she feels comforted and reassured that mother will return. The child has integrated a complex memory of an understanding, reliable, and comforting mother who will return that is triggered by the phrase "be back soon."

The establishment of a therapeutic routine lends predictability and safety and helps to maintain emotional calm. This occurs through the therapist and treating team's continual noncritical acceptance of the patient's feelings combined with a therapeutic dialogue about what specific emotions are being triggered and expressed. In addition, the therapist acknowledges the validity of the patient's emotional response in light of both present and past realities. The therapist, as a keeper of the patient's history, reminds himself or herself and the patient that there are many understandable reasons for the current state of distress based on past history and poor emotional tolerance.

Emotional Expression and Intensification of Affect

Although a long-range goal of treatment with BPD patients is to enable them to identify, label, and tolerate emotional states, in the early stages of treatment patients often complain that they feel worse when they experience and express emotion. The patients have not yet developed effective strategies for soothing themselves, so their emotions are intensely painful and prolonged. Patients will need pragmatic suggestions of activities that will help them calm down. These can include hobbies, walks, meditation, exercise, relaxation exercises, reading, videos, or any activity that has a potentially distracting, nonharmful calming effect. As benign as these suggestions seem, many BPD patients will not readily accept them. As with referrals for medication, they may initially interpret these suggestions as minimizing their problems or pushing away their emotional needs.

Emotional Expression and Attention Seeking

BPD patients do seek attention, often indirectly, through the expression of intense emotions, provocative statements, and dramatic behaviors because they do not know how to be direct and straightforward. The manner in which they express this need is evidence of their poor social skills. At the same time, they may question the reality and legitimacy of their feelings and wonder whether, perhaps, they are merely "seeking attention" as they have been admonished by parents and professionals alike. The treatment team needs to accept that "seeking attention" is legitimate. The therapeutic task is to understand what the patient needs at the moment and help her or him to express these needs more directly. Emotional expression becomes more direct and genuine through acknowledgment of feeling by the treatment team members. Only when affects are mirrored and understood by another do they serve their evolutionary purpose: to determine reasonable and survival-oriented behaviors. Through this process, biologically driven affect becomes biographically based emotion.

Bearing Witness

A central feature of therapeutic work is to sit with and hold the emotional pain of the patient as a parent sits with and holds the crying child. Acknowledgment of how badly the patient feels without the need to "make it better" or provide suggestions or advice is a crucial aspect of effective psychotherapy with BPD patients. This experience enables the patient to feel truly understood and builds emotional endurance and resilience.

Anger

A difficult part of the therapeutic work with BPD patients is focusing on their anger—its presence, origins, and consequences. Patients are often unaware of the pervasiveness of their anger and the extent to which it drives their behavior. Even when the anger is palpable in voice and gesture, patients may not identify it as such. They do not realize how intimidating their anger can appear to others.

As we discussed earlier, anger serves as an "umbrella" emotion within which are mixed states of anger, hurt, disappointment, envy, revenge, and sadness. This helps to explain the intensity of BPD patients' anger and why it can be so frightening and anxiety provoking. They can become emotional terrorists, holding us hostage with both direct and indirect expressions of anger. Treating BPD patients requires a therapist who can tolerate anger, neither personalizing it nor becoming so anxious that she or he is intimidated and coerced by it into premature responses and actions. The therapist has to maintain his or her own emotional equilibrium as he or she is assaulted by the patient's sarcasm, devaluation, and provocative behavior. It can be tempting to fight fire with fire, but this is always a mistake, as BPD patients are akin to kamikaze pilots in their rage. It enables them to maintain control and a sense of honor and blamelessness. They will push to the limits and beyond to maintain their belief system and to save face and a semblance of control. When angry, the patient operates concretely on an "eye for an eye" moral level. The therapist must disengage from any moral battle and work to understand the state that underlies and fuels the anger. This requires identifying each of the other emotions embedded in the anger and their interpersonal precipitants. A concomitant challenge is helping the BPD patient replace anger and rage as a primary motivating force for action in the world. Without this motivation, the patient is often at a loss, because she or he has not learned to act on the basis of what would bring enjoyment.

Moral Development and the Concept of Blame

BPD patients operate at a latency-age level of moral development, where right and wrong are absolutes and moral rectitude carries special power. They are strict judges and set high standards for others, especially those in caregiving and authoritarian positions. Similarly, they work hard themselves to be right and are inordinately sensitive to perceived unjust criticism and blame, many having been raised in a blaming and shaming environment. This makes it difficult for them to see their own role in social situations. They apply a morally dichotomous "right or wrong" analysis to many interpersonal dilemmas. It takes much psychotherapeutic work for them to understand that individuals have competing needs. They are vigilant about the therapist's comments and easily feel blamed. Thus, the therapist often feels as though she or he were walking through a land mine when discussing areas of interpersonal responsibility.

It is important to make a distinction between guilt and blame. Guilt implies remorse over one's action and presupposes the capacity for empathy and a full acceptance of responsibility for what one has done to another. Blame carries a connotation of censure and shaming from one person to another and is developmentally an earlier emotion and interpersonal experience. BPD patients have not developed the capacity to experience guilt fully. Instead, they struggle with an overwhelming fear of the shame and humiliation that they experienced as children. Parents struggling with similar issues often verbally or physically humiliated them for acts of no consequence. The harsh overreaction of caregivers is etched in their mind, and they anticipate it from others.

The development of appropriate guilt occurs by the therapist empathizing, not agreeing, with the patient's point of view for a long period of time. As the patient experiences empathy for herself, she gradually develops empathy for others and can understand how her behavior may be hurtful. Only then can she feel remorse and accept responsibility. The challenge for the therapist is to maintain faith and patience in this reciprocal process. A common fear is that one is colluding with the patient to avoid responsibility and is only compounding the problem. As the patient feels understood by the therapist, she can begin to hear alternative explanations of the behavior and motivation of others that place them in a human and vulnerable light. Eventually, the patient understands her common humanity with others.

Although this developmental step is possible for many BPD patients, it is not possible for all. Those who have more severe dysfunction will never develop full empathic capacity, guilt, and remorse. However, the empathic action of the therapist and treatment team over time decreases their emotional arousal to trigger events and minimizes the degree of interpersonal errors. In the next section, we elaborate further on anger management as it expresses itself through behaviors.

Depression and Anxiety

The comorbidity of BPD with mood disorders is estimated to be 71% (McGlashan et al. 2000). However, even when the disorder is not in an acute state, BPD patients express chronic dysphoria and depression. A valiant effort is required on the part of the therapist to remain hopeful in the face of the patient's tenacious despair, but this is not as heroic a struggle as is required by the patient. Embedded within the patient's chronic depression are years of hurt and hopelessness and a core feeling of being unlovable. The cumulative experience of unmet dependency and affectional needs has built a deep well of desire for emotional support and nurturance. Sometimes only years of experience with the treatment team and use of medications to modulate affective states can start to fill this well. It is only when the patient feels that the well is capable of being filled that chronic depression and despair can be ameliorated. However, depression will still return episodically around interpersonal crises that recreate feelings of blame, helplessness, and self-loathing.

Similarly, BPD patients experience considerable anxiety. This can take the form of acute panic attacks and subthreshold generalized anxiety. Often BPD patients experience aversive tension and dysphoria. When chronic, this dysphoria contributes to substance abuse and addiction and eating disorders. It also underlies many suicide attempts and self-mutilating behaviors (Bohus et al. 2000).

Suicide Thoughts as Obsession

As an expression of chronic dysphoria, many BPD patients are obsessed with thoughts about suicide and ways in which to commit suicide. The obsession ebbs and flows with mood and circumstance but is ubiquitous; it becomes their leitmotif. The obsession develops into a monolithic problem-solving strategy that provides comfort and binds anxiety. BPD patients research methods of suicide with scientific zeal. Their plans can be impressively creative and often devious. Like all obsessions, their preoccupation with suicide can be incredibly resistant to change and, for some, recedes only after years of psychotherapeutic and psychopharmacological treatment.

Within individual therapy, the patient's talk about suicide can be used to monitor their state, as it is often the only way the patient knows how to express feelings. Like the baby's cry, talk of suicide becomes the patient's primary mode for communicating distress. The suicidal state, like anger, is an umbrella state for a variety of emotions arising from interpersonal situations in which the patient feels helpless and alone.

The patient often talks about suicide without fully realizing the impact it has on the therapist. The patient is dissociated from her own emotions and speaks of suicide with *la belle indifférence*. During these times the patient does not feel she is in a relationship with someone who cares about her and will be worried and alarmed by such talk. This creates dissonance for the therapist, who may minimize the potential seriousness because of the patient's seeming absence of affect. To address the dissociation, the therapist must help the patient to experience the therapist in the room as a caring concerned person who will feel terrible if the patient dies. Further, the therapist conveys that the patient's life is valuable and worth living. Through this interchange the therapist points out the patient's dissociation and supplies the missing emotion for the patient. The therapist mirrors empathy the patient should be feeling toward herself. One way of accomplishing this is for the therapist to ask the patient in the session to envision herself as a young child alone with intolerable sadness and hurt and no one to comfort her. The patient usually can find it easier to have empathy from a distance for herself as this small child. The therapist also talks with the patient about how in a dissociated state she can hurt herself because she does not expect that anyone will ever be there to comfort and help her nor will she ever be able to help herself. This kind of transaction may recur throughout the therapy during times of crises.

Over time, the therapist educates the patient about the use of suicide as a monolithic problem-solving strategy. As the patient reports increased suicidal intent, the therapist works with the patient to identify precipitants and differentiate emotional states. For patients who have the capacity for some insight, the therapist helps them to articulate the interpersonal meanings of their specific plans as they relate to present precipitating events and childhood experiences. For patients without capacity for insight, the therapist must determine the current stressors in the environment and provide behavioral and environmental interventions that reduce or eliminate the stressors with the help of a case manager and/or other community support staff. Gradually, as the prosthetic effects of the treatment village provide sufficient containment, suicidality decreases. We will address suicidal attempts and self-mutilating behaviors in the next section.

BEHAVIORAL DYSREGULATION

BPD patients' impaired emotional regulation and inability to describe feelings contributes to their overreliance on behavioral action patterns as a means to both modulate intensity and communicate. Their body remembers its early experience, and they reenact rather than remember. As a result, they are subject to impulsive and/or compulsive responding, which helps to explain the frequency of comorbid diagnoses of eating disorders in women and substance abuse disorders in men (Zanarini et al. 1998).

Impulsiveness

Impulsiveness, defined as unpremeditated action, characterizes the behaviors of BPD patients when they are surprised by intense emotions such as anger or fear. Action follows emotion without mediation through thought and language. These patients are often driven toward an immediate behavioral solution because they cannot tolerate emotional intensity and require immediate relief. Impulsivity originates from a probable genetic and biological vulnerability and an environmentally mediated impaired ability to identify and modulate feeling states.

Compulsive Action Patterns

Often, BPD patients turn toward the compulsive use of a behavior that they have learned decreases or amplifies emotional intensity or to action patterns that have developed layers of interpersonal meaning. BPD patients usually are compulsive in their relationship to pleasurable behaviors such as spending, sex, eating, and drug and alcohol use. These activities serve many functions. They relieve tension, fill up lonely moments, and assuage hurt feelings and quiet anger. The problem for BPD patients is that they are always on the edge, if not over it, of doing serious damage to themselves through these behaviors. They push everything to the limit, lacking an internal barometer for satiation. Enough never quite feels like enough. Also, because BPD patients experience feelings so intensely, it often takes more of everything (e.g., food, alcohol) to calm themselves down.

For some BPD patients, sex has become a behavioral language in which they are fluent. It serves multiple functions as antidepressant, purveyor of need, security blanket, weapon, and means to relieve unbearable anxiety. Both Lillian and Susan in the case histories engaged in promiscuous sex and identified it as a way to dispel dissociative states and feel connected. Although promiscuity can have many destructive health and interpersonal consequences, it may serve as a potentially good prognostic sign, a reaching for a relationship.

We learn to modulate biologically driven behaviors, such as sex, eating, and drinking, within a relationship. They acquire social meanings and serve social functions. Over time, the pleasure gained comes not from the behavior alone but from its being shared with others. The relational aspect helps to modulate the behavior as the well-being experienced from sharing and closeness predominates.

The problem with compulsive behavior is that it loses its social and relational meaning and becomes an end in itself. The behavior becomes a substitute for the missing relationship. Some BPD patients may eat until stuporous and use drugs or drink until they pass out. They may run up large credit card bills and accumulate disastrous debt. The initial pleasure of the behavior is replaced by a drive toward oblivion. As the damaging and painful effects of these behaviors are experienced, the behaviors acquire other meanings and serve other functions. They become a means to punish the self and get back at others. For some, addiction takes over the whole personality and leads to tragic consequences.

It is through the therapeutic relationship and its generalization to relationships with others that BPD patients learn to modulate these behaviors. The first task is to enable the patient to be honest about the behaviors—to talk and learn about their multiple uses. The therapist must realize that these behaviors cannot be relinquished or modified easily. Premature exhortations to stop drinking or join Overeaters Anonymous will be experienced as nonempathic, critical, and judgmental. It is like taking candy from a starving and crying child because the candy lacks proper nutritional value. The child neither knows nor cares about those differences at that moment. The sustaining features of the relationship with the treatment team and therapist and other coping abilities must be developed first. The therapist and treatment team, as the alliance deepens and the supportive nature of the treatment takes effect, help the patient identify what interpersonal events and emotional states trigger the binges. At the same time, team members convey their genuine concern that the behaviors are harmful to the patient's overall welfare. Treatment helps the patient to learn that binges and sprees retard the development of emotional endurance and resilience by avoiding emotions and interfering with the development of more adaptive coping strategies.

As the patient gradually learns what triggers excessive behaviors, the therapist simultaneously encourages alternative activities, such as hobbies, exercise, and meditation, that the patient finds enjoyable. This builds the patient's capacity for pleasure from nondamaging activities. The therapist also encourages the patient to reach out to team members when upset and eventually to friends and supportive family. The patient learns that turning to others who respond compassionately results in regulation of emotion, and this experience reduces and replaces compulsive behaviors. The patient also learns that what she or he is seeking from compulsive behaviors can be found within a supportive relationship or pleasurable activity. Some patients may become compulsive in their use of healthier behaviors, but as long as these behaviors are less damaging, this is preferable to compulsive use of damaging behaviors.

Self-help and recovery groups can be enormously helpful in reinforcing BPD patients' use of adaptive coping skills. These groups reinforce the use of constructive relationships as a means to reduce stress and regulate emotional states. They serve as an extension of the therapeutic relationship and provide a safety net after hours and on weekends. Another important feature of these groups is that they provide a cognitive framework that the patient's experiences as organizing and sustaining.

As discussed earlier in the chapter, a goal of treatment is to help the patient build a village to sustain her or him through the active phases of treatment and beyond. Recovery groups can serve that function for some.

High-Risk Occupations and Hobbies

Some BPD patients, especially males, pursue high-risk occupations and hobbies. They drive fast, take up hobbies such as skydiving, and select work in which their life or others' lives are at stake, such as firefighting or emergency room work. The risk-taking behavior, which is related to their underlying extroverted and high novelty-seeking temperaments, appears to serve a function similar to that served by compulsions and addictions, in that it focuses and calms the patient while helping him or her feel less dissociative and more alive. Through treatment, the patient may continue these activities but learns to take greater precautions and increase safety behaviors.

Substance Abuse

The use of illegal substances is a primary means for many patients, especially males, to regulate emotion, manage dissociation, and cope with interpersonal stressors. Addiction potential may also be part of the genetic vulnerability of BPD patients. Substance dependence was present in three of the four families of BPD patients described in the case histories in this book. Thus, substance abuse is a form of behavioral dysregulation but can become an addiction.

In treating BPD patients with more severe co-occurring disorders, there is a growing body of evidence that integrated treatment is the most effective approach (Drake et al. 1998; Judd et al. 2002; Minkoff 2001a, 2001b). This approach entails provision of psychopharmacological and psychotherapeutic treatment with recovery and relapse prevention methods at one site by cross-disciplinary and cross-trained staff.

Parallel treatment—that is, receiving psychiatric treatment at one site and substance abuse services at another—can be effective for patients with less severe problems and a greater capacity to straddle two systems. However, BPD patients pose special problems when being treated at two sites. The potential for "splitting" is high, and when their manipulative and bullying behaviors are triggered, they are at risk for being ejected from treatment. Thus, both psychiatric and substance abuse treatment providers must work collaboratively to maintain the patient in compliance with needed treatment.

The treatment team may have to facilitate detoxification and residential rehabilitation for BPD patients who are alcohol or substance dependent. The therapeutic relationship should be maintained during periods of detoxification and intensive rehabilitation because the continuity of the relationship helps to maintain sobriety and the motivation to remain sober. If a patient refuses detoxification, more comprehensive methods, such as staged interventions or the threat of loss of the therapeutic relationship, may need to be employed. The latter is used only when the therapist feels no longer able to help the physically addicted patient and can genuinely say that without detoxification the therapy cannot continue. This approach may not work with patients whose addiction has overpowered all will to live, but it is the only and last recourse.

Relapse is an expected part of any recovery process. BPD patients are especially vulnerable to relapse under conditions of high interpersonal stress. The therapist and treatment team can expect that the patient's participation will go through many fits and starts and require continuous encouragement and reinforcement.

Concurrent involvement in Alcoholics Anonymous, Rational Recovery, or other self-help groups can be an important and invaluable adjunct to treatment. However, some patients will refuse group involvement because they suffer from social phobia, have high levels of mistrust and paranoia regarding others, or find groups overwhelming. Not all patients can take advantage of a group format. In these cases, the therapist, after a reasonable effort, is wise to accept the patient's refusal as an indication that self-help groups are not for everyone.

Many patients will continue to abuse substances episodically throughout the course of treatment. The goal is a gradual reduction in the frequency and severity of the use following a harm reduction/risk minimization approach. Some patients will eventually discontinue all substance abuse and use socially, whereas others learn they must quit completely. To insist on abstinence and refuse treatment when a patient does not comply raises a serious ethical problem. There is always hope for the patient as long as she or he maintains the therapeutic relationship and works toward healthier behaviors.

Suicide and Suicidal Behavior

Completed Suicide

The rate of suicide among borderline patients is reported to be between 3% and 10% (McGlashan 1986; Paris et al. 1987; Stone et al. 1987). The presence of impulsive aggression and affective dysregulation appears to be linked with successful suicide (Brent et al., in press). Given the high rate of successful suicide with these patients, the clinician must take talk of suicide very seriously.

As addressed earlier in this chapter, suicidal thinking and behaviors are a persistent and central feature of the disorder and pose many challenges to a treatment team. It is an expression of a core belief that life is not worth living and of ingrained feelings of helplessness and lack of efficacy. As self-murder, suicide represents what many BPD patients feel was done to them psychologically during childhood. For patients who actually feared for their lives as children, suicide is a true enactment of early experience but with the patient now in control of when and how. Suicide is a solution to intolerable suffering and a powerful statement of how their early world failed them.

A main goal of therapy is to keep the patient alive long enough for the treatment alliance to take effect. Early in the therapeutic process, the therapist elicits the patient's suicidal thoughts and plans. Procedures need to be established for times of crisis that outline the therapist and treatment team's availability. We believe it is most helpful to take each suicidal crisis as unique and decide on the form of clinical management that is specific to the current crisis. Early crises in treatment may require hospitalization, whereas later ones may only need an extra session. The therapeutic response shifts over time depending on the needs of the patient. The most effective suicide prevention measure is the strength of the therapeutic bond with the treatment team and the hopefulness engendered by these relationships. The patient also needs to feel continuously connected, contained, and safe.

Suicide Attempts

Suicide attempts are usually made in response to disruptions in important relationships in which the patient feels abandoned, betrayed, or in an intolerable interpersonal dilemma. They may also occur in the context of untreated major depression. The trait of impulsive aggression makes suicide more likely, as does a family history of suicide.

Suicide attempts can also be a form of magical thinking. The action communicates both the desire for resolution, mastery, restoration of self-esteem, and revenge and the hope for rescue, care, reconciliation, and reunion. The action, designed to end all relatedness, is equally designed to restore it. Patients, feeling alone, perform what is meant to be a dyadic interpersonal transaction, ignorant of how to engage in a dialogue about their feelings or assert their needs.

Highly disorganized patients, such as Wendy and Sylvia, are prone to impulsive suicide attempts when overwhelmed. The attempts can occur in response to many different states and circumstances. The patient's intent is to obtain immediate relief, and she will use whatever is readily available, often a combination of pills and alcohol. Use of alcohol may begin as a form of self-medication but escalates and can be lethal or seriously compromise the patient's health.

Unfortunately, but inevitably, severely impaired patients learn that these attempts result in needed relief and care and turn to them doggedly during any crisis. Wendy, as described in Chapter 6, overdosed repeatedly on antipsychotic medicines when unable to cope. Substance abusers are especially vulnerable to impulsive suicide attempts, because alcohol and drugs disrupt basic survival instincts and amplify depression and anger.

Repeated suicide threats and attempts of an impulsive and disorganized nature are a blatant manifestation of serious deficits in affect modulation and problem solving. These recurring threats and attempts reflect greater developmental deviation of both biological and environmental origins and, as such, necessitate a specific treatment response. The patient is communicating a grave disability and telling the treatment team that she or he needs a wider and deeper support system. The patient, in a state of high arousal, needs to feel contained and that she or he has access to continuous support. A 24-hour intensive case management approach with easy access to hospitalization and day treatment is indicated.

The patient's behavior will remain highly unstable and dangerous when access to care is threatened. Hospitalization with medication treatment serves the purpose of calming the patient and restoring equilibrium. Patients who make repeated suicide attempts related to alcohol and drug abuse will also require special substance abuse treatment, as discussed earlier.

Some suicide attempts are a response to perceived betrayal that produces hurt, shame, anger, and a desire for revenge. Anger serves as a powerful motivator for BPD patients and can enable them to mobilize suicide plans. The patient, partially assuming blame for the betrayal and trying to protect the needed relationship, turns the anger on herself or himself. Planning suicide focuses and calms the patient and temporarily lessens her or his distress. The greater the sense of betrayal, the more potentially dramatic the suicide plans, as the patient also seeks revenge. The execution can be dramatic and flamboyant, engaging the attention of a whole community. It is as though the patient wants the world to bear witness to her or his suffering at last. The intent, again, may be not to die but to bring about the needed care from others and to restore a secure attachment. Sadly, many BPD patients die unintentionally, hoping for reunion.

BPD patients who have greater organizational skills are more likely to have the most lethal suicide plans. They bring their intelligence and planning ability to the task. The plan is usually developed in a dissociative state when the patient has lost emotional connection to significant others. In this state, the patient is at great risk as she or he plans the suicide with cool precision. The main goal of the therapy during these times is to reestablish the emotional bond and help the patient to feel reconnected. Once the bond is restored, the precipitants to the suicidal crisis can be understood and the patient's coping can be strengthened.

Suicide and Major Depression

The presence of major depression, especially when the patient is entering into or recovering from a depressive episode, places the patient at higher risk related to greater activation. The patient's problem-solving abilities are more impaired, and her or his sense of isolation is greater. Like all depressed patients, the BPD patient experiences tremendous despair over ever feeling better. However, for BPD patients, who have had considerable real trauma and interpersonal failure, the rationale for suicide appears far more compelling and resistant to cognitive strategies. The depressive cognitive distortions of BPD patients are thus more refractory to therapeutic interventions. What often distinguishes the suicidal talk and plans of the BPD patient from those of patients with major depression alone are the interpersonal import and the trait of impulsivity in the former. Patients with major depression alone generally express more straightforward despair and hopelessness, with suicide being the only means to end their pain. The plans of BPD patients are often convoluted and devious, with greater interpersonal communication, expressing the depth of their despair, longing, rage, and desire for revenge.

Self-Mutilating Behavior

The self-mutilating behavior of BPD patients is reminiscent of the stigmata of early Catholic saints that bore witness to their suffering for Christ. The psychological pain written on the arms and legs of BPD patients bears witness to their suffering in search of a secure attachment to the loved one.

Self-mutilating behavior usually involves cutting oneself with a knife, scissors, or razor blade or burning oneself. The cuts are typically on the inside of the arms, wrists, or upper thighs, where the skin is tender and the cuts can be concealed to the casual observer. The behavior often follows an unbearable prolonged state of dysphoria and anxiety. It also can follow an interpersonal encounter in which the patient felt unjustly blamed and unable to defend herself or himself or deeply misunderstood. However, for some, the behavior can be a response to even minor interpersonal disruptions. Wendy's behavior exemplifies the role of cutting as a response to multiple self states and as a cry for attention.

Unlike a suicide attempt, by which the patient seeks oblivion, self-mutilating behaviors provide temporary relief from suffering through a combination of self-soothing and self-punishment. Recent studies suggest that the relief found in self-mutilation that occurs in a dissociative state may result from the release of endogenous opioid substances mobilized by the self-injury (Bohus et al. 1999, 2000; Leibenluft et al. 1987; Roth et al. 1996; Russ et al. 1994; Winchel et al. 1991). This relief serves as a powerful reinforcement for the continuation of the behavior.

These behaviors are also a potent form of communication. An interpersonal context usually triggers these behavioral enactments of a preverbal schema of hurt, betrayal, and confusion from childhood. The patient, in a dissociated state, re-creates the interpersonal event that just occurred as both actor and the one acted on. The behavior is a concrete expression, a psychological bloodletting, of what the patient feels the other did to her (i.e., cut her to the quick). The patient is saying, "See what you have done to me!" The intent is to get back at the other without acknowledging the anger. At the same time, the patient accepts blame and punishes herself in expiation and throws herself at the mercy of the other, seeking absolution and succor. The patient is engaged in what is meant to be a dyadic transaction, and once the interaction is complete, the patient feels temporary physical and psychological relief and calm.

The manner and extent to which the patient self-mutilates depend on many factors. Some patients cut only in response to highly specific interpersonal conditions, whereas others resort to cutting or its equivalent under all conditions of stress. For some, cutting becomes a separate addictive process, losing its original interpersonal meaning. Cutting can be highly ritualized and elaborate or simple and crude. One patient, Barbara, developed a pattern of injecting anesthetic into her wrists and then systematically cutting as deeply yet as carefully as she could. She studied books on anatomy in the local medical school library to determine how best to perform this self-surgery. Another patient, Jim, cut himself routinely on the chest in intricate patterns. Barbara, tragically, killed herself before the age of 30, and we suspect that the severity and compulsivity of her cutting were signs of a level of disturbance and disorder refractory to available treatment. Of course, there were many other factors contributing to her early death, the chief of which were severe biological vulnerability, childhood maltreatment, and a subsequent inability to sustain any therapeutic or other form of relationship. Marsha Linehan's behavioral treatment for parasuicidal behaviors (Linehan 1993a, 1993b) offers hope for such individuals. Her approach, described in Chapter 7 ("Universal Features of Treatment"), is the only treatment currently available that has outcome data to support its efficacy (Linehan et al. 1993, 1994).

As suggested earlier, patients who use cutting as a generalized stress response tend to be more disabled and require a structured treatment approach aimed at containment and reduction of overall arousal level. Hospitalization, especially brief stays, will do little to treat these phenomena. A treatment option that can be effective but that, unfortunately, is not readily available in most communities is a behavioral modification approach implemented in a long-term residential setting in combination with medications that target anxiety, agitation, and compulsive behavior.

Patients who cut in response to situation-specific stressors may benefit from medications for treatment of acute states and will generally respond to psychotherapeutic strategies. The therapist follows the strategies outlined earlier that help the patient to identify which interpersonal stressors and emotions trigger the cutting and to learn better how to regulate emotion and replace cutting with other behavioral coping strategies.

Anger Enacted Toward the Therapist and Others

BPD patients are extremely sensitive to potential abandonment and a betrayal of trust. They experience panic in the face of abandonment and anger over the betrayal. This combination can lead to impulsive destructive action. Examples include direct action toward the therapist, such as destruction of property and silent, menacing phone calls, or indirect action toward the self, such as threats to jump off a bridge, set oneself on fire, or carry a gun with the intent of provoking the police into shooting them. The extremity of the behavior is a measure of how important the therapeutic relationship is to these patients and how devastated they feel by its disruption.

Because these crises are iatrogenic, they are best managed within the therapeutic relationship when possible. The therapist works to reestablish the therapeutic bond and reassure the patient that the relationship is intact. This may require additional visits and phone contact. The therapist acknowledges his or her part in the therapeutic crisis and "takes the blame" directly and honestly but without self-flagellation. The therapist's ability to accept responsibility is a powerful experience for the patient and usually decreases the intensity of her reaction. It also enables the patient to begin to look at her part in the disruption and to reevaluate her response. The therapist acknowledges how frightened, anxious, and angry the patient must have been to perform such extreme acts that were potentially so harmful to therapist and patient. Further, the therapist suggests that the patient must have reexperienced childhood feelings of powerlessness and abandonment. Alternative ways of coping with such feelings, especially talking instead of acting, are also explored.

When the patient has done damage to property or person, appropriate legal action and reparation is necessary so that others are protected and the patient is held accountable for her or his actions. The treatment team should work with the patient's attorney to achieve an outcome that maximizes the patient's chances of continuing the psychotherapeutic work to the extent possible. The best prevention of future violence is through the provision of consequences and helping the patient understand what led to the eruption of violence and how to manage anger nonviolently.

When a less serious disruption occurs in the therapeutic relationship, the alliance can be renegotiated and repaired with consultation and support. A three-way meeting with therapist, patient, and consultant can be very useful during this process, providing needed support and clarification for all. If the therapist is unable to continue for whatever reason, it is important that the transfer to a new therapist be negotiated carefully.

BPD patients who have severe paranoid, narcissistic, and antisocial features may not be helped by traditional therapeutic methods, and, unfortunately, residential treatment settings that might be more effective do not exist. Thus, patients who exhibit violent behaviors with these features often must be excluded from treatment for the protection of others.

An abrupt ending to a therapeutic relationship is often the most dangerous situation for the patient and therapist. The more abandoned and blamed the patient feels, the greater the potential for more extreme behavior and the more hopeless the patient will feel about ever being helped. It is best if the therapist can convey his or her concern for the patient while, as directly as possible and without the assignation of blame, explaining why he or she feels unable to continue as the therapist. A three-way meeting among patient, therapist, and new therapist and/or with all team members can help to minimize the feeling of abandonment. Hospitalization may also be indicated during this transition. The patient needs to feel held and contained as the transition occurs. Otherwise, fear of abandonment or paranoid anger over betrayal can lead to dangerous and destructive behavior to self and others.

BPD patients usually become dissociated in response to rage and enact their feelings in a seemingly detached and calculated fashion. The plan to hurt and avenge the perceived perpetrator of injustice falls along a continuum from malicious mischief to lawsuits to murder. The more disturbed the patient's thinking, the higher the intelligence, and the greater the degree of cruelty in the patient's childhood, the more potentially disastrous the consequences. For therapeutic purposes, it is important to understand that the patient's analysis of the situation is based on black-and-white thinking, a paranoid distortion of present reality (although not always of the past), and a state of righteousness. The patient loses cognitive flexibility and is unable to empathize with any aspect of the other person's situation. For some patients, the plan springs from years of daydreaming about revenge.

The person to be harmed represents the original abuser. The patient acts as a means to gain mastery over intolerable feelings of helplessness and to right the perceived wrong.

Some patients turn their anger toward abstract victimizers, such as the government, the military, landlords, or big industry. They are spokespersons for the downtrodden and can be vitriolic in their attacks. Although good may come from their efforts, the long-term interpersonal cost is high. Their chronic righteous anger erodes the good will of colleagues and the representatives of the system with whom they interact.

Anger Enacted in the Workplace

In the workplace, individuals with BPD are often extremely hard workers and highly competent, but the interpersonal arena is fraught with potential explosiveness. It replicates an aspect of the parent-child relationship that is especially difficult for the patient. These individuals desperately yearn for recognition and appreciation and often overwork to achieve it. They maltreat themselves through overwork, placing their physical and emotional health at risk. When their efforts are not appreciated, their resentment mounts and angry outbursts or behavior that undermines staff morale can result. Although their work output may be excellent, their attitude can get them into trouble. Their intense demeanor and blunt verbal style can make supervisors and co-workers anxious and wary. They may be hypercritical of others, especially of supervisors, perceiving themselves, in comparison, as working harder and better and being undervalued. Although this perception may be somewhat accurate, it makes co-workers feel intimidated and resentful and results in alienation. BPD patients who have had learning disabilities learned unorthodox work habits that, although effective, are often misunderstood as oppositional and generate negative attention. Finally, individuals with BPD often serve as a bellweather for office discontent and get reputations as troublemakers.

As a result of the above, BPD patients often become embroiled in conflict with supervisors and co-workers that leads to labor-relations suits and workmen's compensation battles. The therapeutic challenge is to stay on the patient's side while gradually helping the patient to see her role in the conflict. The therapist, through recognizing and validating the patient's hard work and good intentions, identifies the anger and hurt that underlies her troublesome interactions. The patient has to learn to see herself as others see her when she is angry. The fact that others are intimidated and upset by the patient usually comes as an enormous shock, so stuck is she in her view of herself as helpless victim.

When anger is combined with a paranoid state, BPD patients can be dangerous. There are tragic instances we have witnessed in clinical practice and read of in the daily news of BPD patients who have killed another when in a paranoid or dissociated state and/or under the influence of drugs or alcohol. In these circumstances, of course, the criminal justice system takes over completely, and remaining family are assisted in obtaining services as needed.

FINAL COMMENTS

We end our discussion of treatment with the words of the Chestnut Lodge patients presented here, as only our patients can truly educate us about what is effective. Lillian recalled the structure that allowed her to rearrange her thought processes and put together a "jigsaw puzzle of her life so as to determine her own views." The strength of her therapist and his ability to keep her from "veering too far" were also essential. Finally, she emphasized her own motivation as a key factor and the opportunity to experience success in hospital activities.

Susan felt that treatment at Chestnut Lodge provided her with a foundation. She especially valued her experience with a female hospital aide who "let me be myself" and could handle her emotional swings. Finally, she celebrated her therapist, who helped her to learn about herself and made the difference between "mere existence and a meaningful life."

Sylvia, because of her untimely death, was unable to articulate her thoughts on her treatment at Chestnut Lodge, although she did indicate to her last therapist that she felt she had made "good progress" while there. Her decision to live close to the hospital where she was first treated suggests that she understood and accepted her need for an ongoing secure attachment to a system of care that replaced her own disorganized attachment system. She created her own village, and within a few blocks of her home she had access to her psychiatrist/therapist, the hospital, the AA community, the art community, and a variety of potential live-in aides.

Wendy, befitting her greater impairment, was less articulate but stated ardently that while she disliked the seclusion and restraint, her therapist and the treatment at Chestnut Lodge were the best in her 30 years of treatment, contrasting with the "barbaric" treatment she experienced elsewhere. She recalled how close she felt to her Chestnut Lodge therapist, even after 15 years of absence. Wendy's testimony suggests that, as Ezra Pound, who spent many years hospitalized at St. Elizabeth's psychiatric hospital in Washington, D.C., wrote, "nothing matters but the quality of affection in the end that leaves its trace in the mind."

REFERENCES

Adler G, Buie PH: Aloneness and borderline psychopathology: the possible relevance of child development issues. Int J Psychoanal 60:83–96, 1979

Bohus MJ, Landwehrmeyer GB, Stiglmayr CE, et al: Naltrexone in the treatment of dissociative symptoms in patients with borderline personality disorder: an open-label trial, J Clin Psychiatry 60:598–603, 1999

Bohus M, Limberger M, Ebner U, et al: Pain perception during self-reported distress and calmness in patients with borderline personality disorder and self-mutilating behavior. Psychiatry Res 95:251–260, 2000

Brent DA, Oquendo M, Birmaher B, et al: Familial pathways to early onset suicide attempt: a high-risk study. Arch Gen Psychiatry (in press)

Damasio A: The Feeling of What Happens. New York, Harcourt Brace, 1999

Drake E, Merer-McFadden C, Mueser K, et al: Review of integrated mental health and substance abuse treatment for patients with dual disorders. Schizophr Bull 24:589–603, 1998

Gunderson JG: The borderline patient's intolerance of aloneness, insecure attachments, and therapist availability. Am J Psychiatry 153:752–758, 1996

Judd P, Thomas N, Hough RL: UCSD/San Diego County Dual Diagnosis Demonstration Project: a prospective study of long-term outcomes and cost benefits. Poster presentation at the Academy of Health Services Research and Health Policy Annual Research Meeting, Washington, DC, June 25, 2002

Lane RD, Schwartz GD: Levels of emotional awareness: a cognitive-developmental theory and its application to psychopathology. Am J Psychiatry 144: 133–143, 1987

Leibenluft E, Gardner DL, Cowdry RW: The inner experience of the borderline self-mutilator. Journal of Personality Disorders 1:317–324, 1987

Linehan MM: Cognitive-Behavioral Treatment of Borderline Personality Disorder. New York, Guilford, 1993a

Linehan MM: Skills Training Manual for Treating Borderline Personality Disorder. New York, Guilford, 1993b

Linehan MM: Understanding Borderline Personality Disorder. New York, Guilford, 1995

Linehan MM, Heard HL, Armstrong HE: Naturalistic follow-up of a behavioral treatment for chronically parasuicidal borderline patients. Arch Gen Psychiatry 50:971–974, 1993

Linehan MM, Tutek DA, Heard HL, et al: Interpersonal outcome of cognitive behavioral treatment for chronically suicidal borderline patients. Am J Psychiatry 151:1771–1776, 1994

McGlashan T: The Chestnut Lodge Follow-Up Study, Part III: long-term outcome of borderline personalities. Arch Gen Psychiatry 42:20–30, 1986

McGlashan TH, Grilo CM, Skodol AE: The Collaborative Longitudinal Personality Disorders Study: baseline Axis I/II and II/II diagnostic co-occurrence. Acta Psychiatr Scand 102:256–264, 2000

Minkoff K: Developing standards of care for individuals with co-occurring psychiatric and substance use disorders. Psychiatr Serv 52:597–599, 2001a

Minkoff K: Program components of a comprehensive integrated care system for seriously mentally ill patients with substance disorders. New Dir Ment Health Serv 91:17–30, 2001b

Paris J, Brown R, Nowlis D: Long-term follow-up of borderline patients in a general hospital. Compr Psychiatry 28:530–535, 1987

Roth AS, Ostroff RB, Hoffman RE: Naltrexone as a treatment for repetitive self-injurious behavior: an open-label trial. J Clin Psychiatry 57:233–237, 1996

Russ MJ, Roth SD, Kakuma T, et al: Pain perception in self-injurious borderline patients: naloxone effects. Biol Psychiatry 35:207–209, 1994

Stone MH, Hurt SW, Stone DK: The P.I.-500: long-term follow-up of borderline in-patients meeting DSM-III criteria, I: global outcome. Journal of Personality Disorders 1:291–298, 1987

Winchel RM, Stanley M: Self-injurious behavior: a review of the behavior and biology of self-mutilation. Am J Psychiatry 148:306–317, 1991

Zanarini MC, Frankenburg FR, Dubo ED, et al: Axis I comorbidity of borderline personality disorder. Am J Psychiatry 155:1733–1739, 1998

Index

Page numbers printed in **boldface** *type refer to figures.*